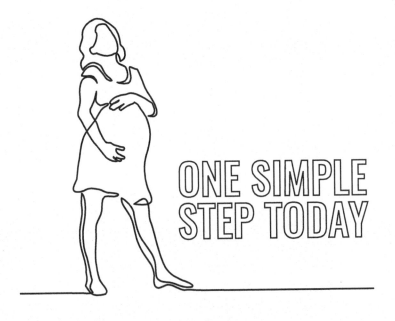

ONE SIMPLE STEP TODAY

Connecting With Your Body Throughout Pregnancy

Heather Marra, PT

DISCLAIMER

This book is not intended to diagnose or prescribe any treatment for any medical or psychological conditions. It is not to replace medical treatment. This book contains the ideas and opinions of its author and is intended to provide helpful and educational information.

The individual reading this book should continue medical care with appropriate healthcare providers and seek their approval before adopting any suggestions in this book.

To Pete, my husband,
Encouraging me to take One Simple Step Today;
Without you, this would still be a dream.

To Peter, Mateja, and Max,
You breathe joy into every part of my life.

TABLE OF CONTENTS

PAIN IS COMMON,
BUT PAIN IS
not normal.

INTRODUCTION

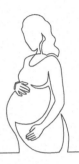

One Simple Step Today was created for busy women who don't need another "To Do" on their list, but who want to take steps toward a healthy and strong pregnancy. Congratulations on taking a step today! By purchasing this book, you have already taken a step toward a healthier YOU. You will find links to videos throughout the book to help with learning and provide greater understanding.

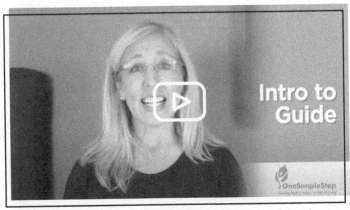

Intro to Guide

OneSimpleStep

Click to view video or view full link listing at the end of the chapter.

As a mom of three children and a physical therapist, I know what it is like to have a busy schedule. Between work, family, friends, errands, and responsibilities, who needs to add an extra pregnancy workout or long, confusing grocery list to her already full day?

This book, along with all other *One Simple Step Today* plans, is designed to help you move toward a healthier and more fit pregnancy AS YOU GO ABOUT YOUR DAY. It's not an extra thing to do, but rather it's a guide for moving well and listening to your body throughout the regular course of your day.

As a pelvic floor physical therapist, my passion is to help women find wholeness, healing, and freedom. We as women help so many others, but we often neglect ourselves.

In a 2018 study, up to 86 percent of surveyed pregnant women reported pelvic girdle pain and/or low back pain. Only 24 percent of these women in the U.S. received treatment. Of all the women who did receive treatment, 68 to 87 percent reported a positive effect.[i]

The take-home message here is that pregnancy-related pain is common. Many women do not seek out treatment. When women did seek out help, there was a great improvement in their symptoms during pregnancy.

How about you? I hope through learning more about your body during pregnancy and beyond, that you can speak up for yourself and ask for support or treatment when you face a physical or emotional obstacle. You do have options! Pain is common, but pain is never normal.

Pregnancy is not just another chapter in our lives…it is a very important chapter and one where we can either make bad habits worse or make the decision to live with intention.

During pregnancy, our weak areas shine brightly. As we carry the extra load of pregnancy, movement that was once just irritating can become downright painful. The worst part is that people often tell us that the pain is normal, okay, or even to be expected! Let me reassure you that pain is common during pregnancy, but it should not be dismissed as normal. Neither should it be ignored. When you learn how to move in ways that support your pelvic floor and your back, you can confidently move with intention. This intentional care for your body leads to a more pain-free life during, and after, your pregnancy.

I have been a firsthand witness to what happens when women ignore pain or discomfort. It often begins as early as childhood! After 20 years as a physical therapist, I cannot tell you how many women have told me one of the following things:

"As a child, I occasionally didn't make it to the toilet to use the bathroom."

or

"I peed a little when I ran when I was a kid."

or

"My parents told me I had a tiny bladder."

These minor concerns were ignored. The reason these women ignored their pelvic floor issues, even as a child, is because their mother or aunt or grandmother or friend told them, "Don't worry about it! This is completely normal. It happens to me, too!"

That same child continues to have problems in adolescence. Teenage girls make statements like:

"Teachers think I am trying to get out of class because I have to go every hour."

or

"Every now and then, I pee a little when I play volleyball."

Fast forward to pregnancy. Now, this same girl who used to pee a little when she ran has a baby resting on her bladder. She now begins to leak when she coughs, sneezes, or lifts a heavy load. During a time when she was looking forward to tossing out the pads, she begins wearing a pad regularly.

I want to help these women understand,

YOU HAVE A PELVIC FLOOR, BUT YOU NEED TO LEARN ABOUT IT, HOW IT FUNCTIONS, AND HOW TO STRENGTHEN IT.

But unfortunately, most women do not see a physical

therapist during their pregnancy. Even their doctors tell them, "This is completely normal. Don't worry!"

In other countries, like France, it is a requirement for a woman to see a physical therapist at 6-week postpartum to assess her pelvic floor, scar tissue, and abdominals and core for strength and coordination tips before returning to exercise, sex, and normal life routines.[ii]

However, that kind of support is not a standard of care in the USA. In fact, that is one of the reasons I am writing this book. I want women to know that these kinds of problems do not have to be the norm for them. They do not have to accept pain as normal and continue with habits that are exacerbating the problem.

Let's continue with this same scenario. After giving birth, the woman who peed when she ran as a child, and wore a pad during pregnancy, will likely begin to leak a little when she exercises. Then, as a young mom, she might report the following to her friends:

"You know, I cannot even jump on the trampoline with my kids."

or

"I wear a pad when I play tennis."

The other moms shrug their shoulders and say, "These kids have ruined our bodies!"

As this same woman gets older, she begins wearing a thicker pad almost every day. This point of discomfort is when she makes an appointment with someone like me. She is fifty-five and is tired of dealing with this issue.

I have good news and bad news for this woman. The good news is that we can take simple steps today to strengthen her body and relieve her discomfort. The bad news is she could have taken these steps when she was a child and avoided all of it.

This scenario is just ONE example of how a small, seemingly insignificant problem can continue throughout a woman's life, including during pregnancy.

It is important to know that although a symptom may be common, it is not normal. One study showed that a third of women have urinary incontinence (UI) and up to one-tenth have fecal incontinence (FI) after childbirth. [iii] Incontinence is the unwanted loss or leakage of poop or pee. Never should incontinence be seen as a normal part of aging or consequence of pregnancy.

I have written this book so you can take simple steps each day to move with intention during your pregnancy. My goal is for you to see your health during this time of your life as part of your overall lifelong health. You might be bringing some unhealthy habits into your pregnancy, but during this time, if they are not corrected, they will intensify. The good news is, they can be corrected now to set you up for a lifetime of holistic care for yourself. It is a domino effect, so let's start knocking over some healthy, happy dominos that will serve your overall health for years to come!

Often, pregnant women say, "My goal is healthy mom and healthy baby." Let's raise the bar higher. Your health is not just physical, but emotional, mental, and spiritual. The focus is not just getting to the delivery. May this time during your pregnancy be a preparation for not just delivery, but your postpartum life and years to come.

So, take time each day to prepare for delivery, healthy postpartum, and a healthy life by going through one chapter per day.

You will find video links throughout the book. This bonus content will make it easier to understand and apply the tips and techniques discussed in each chapter. Go to: www.onesimplestep.today/bookvideos. Enter your information and the videos will be emailed to you.

Throughout this book, I mention that during and after pregnancy essential oils can be helpful throughout the day to reduce anxiety, promote better sleep, reduce lower back pressure, and promote overall wellbeing. There are many brands available and many levels of quality. Personally, I use and highly recommend the Young Living Essential Oil brand. They are of high therapeutic quality and women consistently receive comforting results with this brand. For more information: www.onesimpleoil.today.

INTRODUCTION VIDEO LINK

Video #1: Introduction to the Guide
www.onesimplestep.today/bookvideos

Journal & Reflection

DO I SEE PAIN AS NORMAL? HOW DO I VIEW PAIN?

_____

_____

_____

_____

_____

_____

WHAT HEALTHY HABITS AM I BRINGING INTO MY PREGNANCY?

_____

_____

_____

_____

_____

_____

_____

_____

IN WHAT AREAS IN MY LIFE DO I WANT MORE WHOLENESS, HEALING OR FREEDOM?

_____

_____

_____

_____

_____

_____

_____

_____

_____

_____

_____

_____

_____

THERE IS NO CORE
WITHOUT
the pelvic floor.

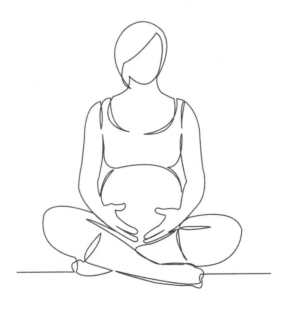

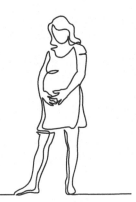

DAY 1

KNOW YOUR BODY

Let's knock down an important domino first. Before we can accurately listen to our bodies, exercise our bodies, and even correctly feed our bodies, we need to really know our bodies. It's time to learn about your anatomy!

As you prepare for pregnancy and childbirth, there is never a better time to complete your education in YOU. Why is today the perfect day to take one small step toward a healthier, happier, more educated YOU?

- If you experience pain or discomfort during your pregnancy, it is critical to be able to pinpoint the location and source of that pain. That is pretty tough when you are using phrases like, "It hurts down there."

- Every person has a different "normal." Reading books with diagrams is a start, but today, you are not just going to identify muscles and bones in a book. You are going to take time to locate those body parts on yourself. By observing each part when it is healthy, you will more quickly identify when something has gone awry.

- When you're in birthing classes, you will be able to understand more clearly the instructions you are receiving. You will get more out of your prenatal visits and classes by starting with a strong base of understanding about your body.

- Giving birth is often called a marathon or a gymnastics class. By becoming aware of your body, you can prepare well and understand exactly what nurses and doctors are saying. It will give you peace of mind and confidence as you prepare for delivery.

- Sex is better when you know your body! You can communicate clearly with your partner and gain insight that improves your sex life.

- And finally, you will be able to pass on this understanding to the baby you will be birthing soon. As you become more educated about your own body, you will be a better parent and role model for the child you are lovingly carrying now.

And so, I congratulate you once again on taking an important step today. You are taking a step that will impact your whole body, whole life, and whole family. It is a step toward wholeness!

WHAT IS THE PELVIC FLOOR AND WHY IS IT IMPORTANT?

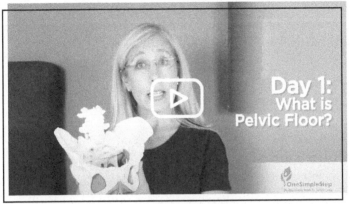

Click to view video or view full link listing at the end of the chapter.

Let's begin our anatomy lesson with a group of muscles called the "pelvic floor."

Your pelvic floor is multiple layers of muscles that are dynamic and help control your three holes—the urethra (to prevent leakage of urine), the vaginal opening (for sexual function and to help support and prevent pelvic organ prolapse and pelvic floor pressure), and anus (to prevent leakage of gas or stool).

Why are we starting with the pelvic floor? Shouldn't we begin with the uterus? This is a pregnancy guide, right?

Yes, your uterus will grow 500 times its normal size in pregnancy, and where does that uterus sit? It sits on your pelvic floor!

The pelvic floor is in the center of our bodies. It absorbs pressure and forces going from the top of the body downward as well as pressure and forces from the legs up. These layers of muscles must be working together in order for you to use the restroom, enjoy sex, and have a successful vaginal birth, as well as assisting with all the movements you complete throughout a day.

Luckily, these muscles work without us having to even think about them, most of the time. Sometimes, and often during pregnancy, the pelvic floor becomes dysfunctional. This problem can lead to various types of pelvic pain, leakage of urine or stool or gas, or pelvic organ prolapse (uterus, bladder, or rectum drops from its normal position).

Unfortunately, it is estimated that 1 in 3 women will experience incontinence at some time in their lives.[iv] So, even though you picked up this book as a pregnancy guide, my hope is that it will not only help you identify and prevent pain during pregnancy but also identify and prevent other disruptions throughout your lifetime.

This may be the first time you have had to consider the pelvic floor. Or you might sail through pregnancy symptom-free and then one day think, "Everything has changed." We don't want to accept changes as the new norm. This is not to instill fear. Rather, it is to give hope through education. We have so much potential that we don't want to be derailed by pain or discomfort.

The pelvic floor must be able to perform three distinct tasks to function properly. It must be able to:

- Contract or Elevate or Lift
- Relax
- Lengthen

However, because most women don't know what the pelvic floor is, they don't take care to strengthen, relax, and coordinate these muscles with the demands of the day. They also do not recognize early signs of dysfunction, waiting until it's very painful or they experience symptoms of leaking or pressure to seek treatment.

This lack of understanding keeps women from accurately listening when their bodies are talking to them. They ignore signs and write them off as normal, or they become consumed by the pain and paralyzed by fear, especially during pregnancy.

My goal is to help you LIVE WITH FREEDOM.

Let me introduce the core. It's more than just abdominals. The core is like a box. Think about the top being the diaphragm. The front is the abdominals. The bottom of the box is the pelvic floor. The back of the box is the back muscles.

The pelvic floor dynamically moves every time you take a breath. If you think of your core as a balloon, you can imagine the process of expansion as air enters the lungs. As we inhale, the lungs fill with air as the diaphragm comes down. This movement should cause the pelvic floor to expand downward as well. As we exhale, the pelvic floor recoils back up.

HOW DOES THE PELVIC FLOOR MOVE?

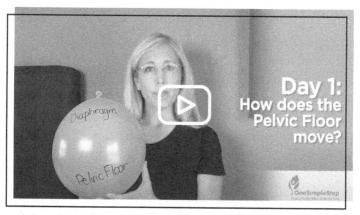

Click to view video or view full link listing at the end of the chapter.

The core can become dysfunctional by sucking in your tummy, holding in your belly button, overworking your abs, or exercising improperly. If you are not breathing correctly, it can also be a hindrance.

Now, add pregnancy to incorrect movement and breathing, and you can see the potential for unwanted symptoms. As the pregnancy progresses, the uterus grows, the belly expands, and everything begins to get tight in the abdominal area. As a result of decreased movement, it is easy to lose rib mobility in pregnancy. If you lose mobility of your ribs, then the pressure transfers to the abdominal wall or the pelvic floor. Everything gets out of whack quickly!

The end results can be:

- Incontinence (unwanted loss of urine or stool)
- Pelvic organ prolapse (uterus, bladder, or rectum drops from its normal position)
- Diastases recti (separation of abdominal muscles)
- Back pain
- Pelvic pain

Due to the uterus and baby growing, there will be different pressures in the abdominal area and core. With this changing center of gravity, the intra-abdominal pressure moves toward your weakest point. The result can be imbalance and dysfunction or pain. The balance of your internal system is shifting and changing every day in pregnancy.

Now that you have spent time learning about your pelvic floor, you have given yourself a gift that will last a lifetime. You have begun learning about the core, and that will affect your life each and every day.

Your *One Simple Step Today* is to begin listening to your body, celebrate your body, and have gratitude for everything your body does every day for you—all the amazing parts that function without you even thinking about it!

Journal & Reflection

I AM GRATEFUL FOR MY BODY. IT IS AMAZING THAT MY BODY DOES:

_____

_____

_____

_____

_____

IF I STOPPED AND LISTENED TO MY BODY, IT WOULD TELL ME:

_____

_____

_____

_____

_____

_____

_____

_____

DAY 1 VIDEO LINKS

What is the Pelvic Floor?
www.onesimplestep.today/bookvideos

How Does the Pelvic Floor Move?
www.onesimplestep.today/bookvideos

THE AREA
'down there'
HAS SPECIFIC
NAMES AND PARTS!

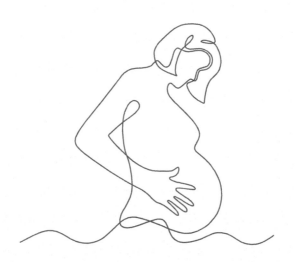

DAY 2

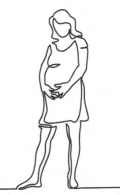

ANATOMY: BONES, MUSCLES, AND PELVIC FLOOR

Often, I hear people refer to the area "down there." Others have nicknames and are embarrassed to use the correct names. This could be a result of upbringing, culture, or just not taking the time to learn. "I'm not in the medical field" is another excuse. Others are too overwhelmed by the complexity.

Let's learn about what bones and muscles are working together to keep your body working properly. Today, we will identify the body parts with correct names and learn about their functions.

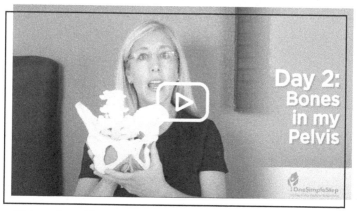

Click to view video or view full link listing at the end of the chapter.

PELVIC GIRDLE – A basin-shaped complex of bones that connects the trunk and the legs, supports and balances the trunk, and contains and supports the intestines, rectum, bladder, and the reproductive organs.

ASIS – The Anterior Superior Iliac Spine (abbreviated: ASIS) is a bony projection of the iliac bone and an important landmark of the pelvis. It refers to the front of the pelvis, which provides attachment for muscles and ligaments.

 Put your hands on your hips. Now, follow the bone forward. The bony part that faces forward is your ASIS.

PUBIC SYMPHYSIS – The joint that sits between and joins the left and right sides of the pelvis. It is located in front and below the bladder. It's the anterior (front) landmark for the pelvic floor.

 Start at your belly button and go down until you feel the bony area. This is the pubic symphysis.

ISCHIAL TUBEROSITY OR "SIT BONES" – As a pair, the sit bones are located at the bottom of the pelvis. It marks the lateral (side) boundary of the pelvic floor and the pelvic outlet, which is important during delivery.

Check now. Are you sitting on your sit bones? If you are slouched, then the answer is no. Sit tall...can you feel the bones under your butt in contact with the chair? Also, try to feel them with you hand. Put your hand under your butt...feel the bony points on the right and left side?

COCCYX – Also known as the tailbone, it is a small, triangular bone resembling a shortened tail located at the bottom of the spine. This bone moves during delivery to open the pelvic outlet. It is also the posterior (back) landmark of the pelvic floor.

Put your hand on your back and continue down toward the "tip of your tail." You may feel it drop off. This is the coccyx. If you continue, you will come to your anus, or rectal opening.

SACRUM – A shield-shaped bony structure that is located at the base of the lumbar vertebrae and is connected to the pelvis. The sacrum forms the posterior (back) pelvic wall and strengthens and stabilizes the pelvis. The sacrum sits above the tailbone.

SI JOINTS – The Sacroiliac Joint is located between the iliac bones and the sacrum, connecting the spine to the hips. The two joints provide support and stability and play a major role in absorbing impact when walking and lifting. From the back, the SI joints are located below the waist where two dimples are visible.

 Put your hands on your hips and slide your hands back toward your butt. You will find a bony area, which then dips in. This is the SI joint. If you look in the mirror, you will see the dimples.

LUMBAR VERTEBRAE – Five vertebral bones with discs between that form the spine in the lower back. These vertebrae carry all of the upper body's weight while providing flexibility and movement to the trunk region.

 Feel your back. Do you feel the bumps in the center? These are the lumbar vertebrae.

ILIAC CREST – The crest of the ilium is the superior or top border of the wing of the ilium and the top of the pelvis.

 Go back to standing with your hands on your hips. Yes, you are on your iliac crest! They are also called the wings of the pelvis.

RIBS – Long curved bones which form the rib cage, part of the bony skeleton. The ribs surround the chest, enabling the lungs to expand and thus facilitate breathing by expanding the chest cavity.

 Just under your bra strap, place your hands around your trunk. These are your ribs. Try it right now. Inhale

through your nose like you're smelling the roses. Do you feel the ribs expand in all directions? It's like an umbrella opening up.

MUSCLES OF THE CORE

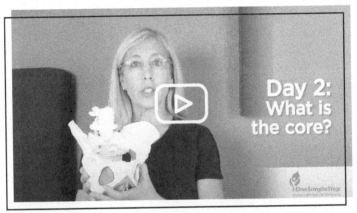

Click to view video or view full link listing at the end of the chapter.

Remember, there is no core without a pelvic floor. Core is a popular word. But what is it exactly? Is it just another name for abs?

Your core is so much more! It is the center of all your movements. With your core you can become more balanced and stronger and more stable. It is always important, but more now in your pregnancy and postpartum than ever before.

Remember, the core can be described as a box.

Diaphragm is the top, abdominals are the front, back muscles are the back, and pelvic floor is the bottom. Let's dig a little deeper to understand more.

TRANSVERSE ABDOMINIS – A deep abdominal muscle layer that runs left and right. It is part of the abdominal wall but is deep to (layered below) the internal/external oblique muscle and rectus abdominus.

 Put your hands on your ASIS (front bony area of your pelvis). Slide off the bone and slightly toward your belly button. Inhale, exhale and feel this area tighten? Sometimes the transverse abdominis is called the corset muscle.

PELVIC FLOOR MUSCLES – Wrapped like a figure eight around your three holes, they form a bowl between your pubic bone, tail bone, and sit bones. You may read in articles or hear about the Levator Ani, which is the deepest layer of pelvic floor muscles: puborectalis, pubococcygeus, and iliococcygeus.

We'll discuss these more, and I will share several tips on how to turn these muscles, on Day #4. You can skip there now if you're curious!

MULTIFIDUS – A very thin muscle, deep in the spine. It works to stabilize the joints at each segmental level. The stiffness and stability make each vertebra work more effectively. The plural of multifidus is multifidi.

 Feel the vertebrae in your lower back, the bony part that sticks out. Slide your fingers off on either side of the bone and you will feel the multifidi along with erector spinae paraspinals (another back muscle). Arch your back and feel the muscles tighten; round your back and feel the muscles relax.

DIAPHRAGM – The largest and strongest muscle in the body. It is dome-shaped and divides the thoracic cavity (containing heart and lungs) from the abdomen. It is essential to breathing. It automatically contracts and relaxes with breathing. Inhale, and this muscle contracts, which causes downward movement and allows for expansion of the lungs and rib cage. Exhale, and it returns to its resting state.

Put your hands on your ribs and breathe in and out. Feel the ribs move? Feel air fill your lungs? This is possible because of your amazing diaphragm that keeps you breathing without even thinking about it!

It's true, there's more to your core than abs!

"WHAT'S DOWN THERE?"
Functional Anatomy of Vagina and Vulva

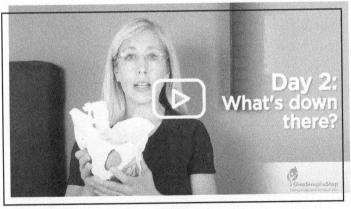

Click to view video or view full link listing at the end of the chapter.

Today, we are also going to identify the parts of your functional anatomy. This portion of self-understanding is important for your journey toward delivery, parenthood, and wholeness. However, after helping women on this journey for twenty years, I know this can be traumatic for many women for many reasons.

First, culturally and religiously, every person has been brought up differently. This is truly a private area of your body, and you may have been taught to view it in a variety of ways. From celebration to shame to abuse, every woman has experienced her own personal journey.

On this day, we are going to get to know our bodies better so we can live a life where we best care for ourselves. However, this may trigger a range of emotions. If you feel the need to speak with a counselor before or after this day, I encourage you to take that step. This is all part of the healing we experience as we become mothers. It is important that we heal our wounds rather than unknowingly passing them on to our children.

However, as a physical therapist, I am going to focus on your physical health and take you on a journey to explore your physical body. If you experience emotional symptoms, then reach out to a licensed counselor or therapist as well.

Let's begin. Get a handheld mirror so you can learn about your body. Your body is unique. Becoming familiar with your body is so important.

Close the door, so you have privacy. With the mirror, you can stand with one foot on the toilet. Another option is sitting on the bed, with your back against the headboard; you may have to use your fingers to open the skin folds so you can see more easily. The skin folds are the labia majora and labia minora.

VULVA – The area women commonly call their vagina. However, the outer area between pubic bone and anus is called the vulva. This is the area that touches your underwear. The internal area is the vagina.

MONS PUBIS – The fatty tissue area above the pubic bone, where pubic hair grows.

LABIA MAJORA – Also can be described as the outer lips of the vulva. This area also has hair growth.

LABIA MINORA – Inside the labia majora are the inner lips of the vulva. There is no hair on this area. The labia minora protects the vagina. Sometimes the labia minora is bigger than the labia majora. Every woman is unique. It's important that you know what's normal for you.

CLITORIS – A small mass of erectile tissue in the female that is situated at the anterior (front) of the vulva, near the meeting of the labia majora (vulvar lips). What is visible is technically called the clitoral glans and is covered by the clitoral hood. There is "more beneath the surface" regarding the clitoris, as 90% of it is internal. The shape of the clitoris actually resembles a wishbone. Like the penis, the clitoris is highly sensitive to stimulation during sex. The sole purpose of the clitoris is for sexual enjoyment.

URETHRA – The tube and opening that leads from the bladder and transports and discharges urine outside the body.

VAGINA – The opening of the vagina is called the vaginal vestibule or introitus. It's located between the urethra and the anus. This opening is where menstrual blood leaves the body and where you insert a tampon. The vaginal cavity is also used to birth a baby and for sexual intercourse. The vaginal cavity is inside the vaginal opening. Above the vaginal cavity is the cervix, which is the bottom part of the uterus. The uterus is where the fetus grows. During pregnancy, the placenta is also inside the uterus.

ANUS – Opening where the gastrointestinal tract ends and exits the body. The anus starts at the bottom of the rectum, the last portion of the colon. This is where poop (stool) leaves the body during a bowel movement.

PERINEAL BODY – Also known as the perineum. The area between the vaginal opening and anus. This is the area where a tear or episiotomy (surgical incision to perineum) may occur in a vaginal delivery.

Your journey through pregnancy is beautiful in so many ways. It forces you to get to know this part of your body better and for many of you, it will provide an opportunity for you to heal, process emotions, and even connect with your partner.

As you continue on this path toward holistic healing, remember that this will carry on for the remainder of your life. You have taken an important step today in your lifetime journey of health. You may need to repeat this exercise more than once in order to feel confident about each term you have learned today.

Your improved education level has ripple effects in your family and even your circle of friends. You will now be able to give better advice, have better conversations, and know when to ignore bad advice.

As you're getting ready to take a shower or undress, your *One Simple Step Today* is to look at yourself and become more familiar with your body. Your body is beautifully made!

DAY 2 VIDEO LINKS

My Pelvic Bones
www.onesimplestep.today/bookvideos

What Is the Core?
www.onesimplestep.today/bookvideos

What's Down There?
www.onesimplestep.today/bookvideos

Journal & Reflection

THINKING BACK ON MY CHILDHOOD, THESE WERE SOME THINGS I WAS TAUGHT ABOUT MY BODY:

_____

_____

_____

_____

_____

WOW, I LEARNED MORE ABOUT MY BODY "DOWN THERE". I DIDN'T REALIZE THAT :

_____

_____

_____

_____

_____

_____

_____

_____

AS I READ THROUGH THIS CHAPTER, I EMOTIONALLY FELT:

(If this is a lot to process, speaking with a therapist/counselor may be very helpful)

_____

_____

_____

_____

_____

_____

_____

_____

_____

_____

_____

_____

_____

WE
breathe and function
WITHOUT PAYING
ATTENTION TO
THE HOW!

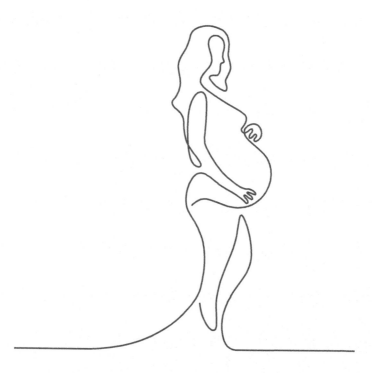

DAY 3

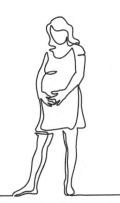

DIAPHRAGMATIC BREATHING

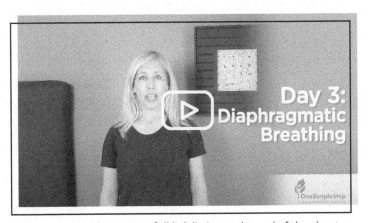

Click to view video or view full link listing at the end of the chapter.

Breathing is one of the many complex and amazing things our bodies do without much thought. We just breathe. Unless you have taken a yoga class or a singing lesson, you probably have not been taught to do this well. Unfortunately, over time, you can develop dysfunctional or paradoxical breathing patterns, muscle restriction, or bad posture as a result of not developing this skill. Consequently, your current breathing patterns become your new normal, but normal does not mean optimal.

Most of us "shallow breathe" during a large percentage of the day. Shallow breathing uses the top one third of our lungs and does not engage the full capacity of our lungs. When taking a shallow breath, our shoulders rise and fall, not allowing the air to fill the lungs and expand the lower part of our core. The result of constant shallow breathing is paradoxical or dysfunctional breathing. Breathing this way can contribute to tightness in the neck and shoulders, chronic muscle tension and even lead to headaches.

However, we can combat shallow breathing with daily diaphragmatic breathing. This practice is not just "belly breathing." It is the type of deep breathing that causes your ribs to expand outward. If you place your hands around your ribs and stand in front of the mirror, you are able to feel and see your ribs expand. This is often referred to as "360-degree breathing." While you are there, check to make sure your shoulders stay in place.

Another way to think about Diaphragmatic Breathing is to count:

- Inhale for 4 seconds.
- Hold for 2 seconds.
- Exhale for 4 to 6 seconds.
- Pause for 2 seconds.

As you inhale, both your ribs and belly should expand. Don't forget the ribs! It is easy to just breathe into your belly, but you want more than just belly breathing. If you place one hand on your belly and one on your ribs, you should feel both expand. Think of your rib cage like an umbrella that is opening thoroughly.

IT IS BEST TO BEGIN DIAPHRAGMATIC BREATHING EARLY IN PREGNANCY SO YOU CAN ENJOY THE BENEFITS THROUGHOUT ALL THREE TRIMESTERS.

Here are different positions you can begin to practice diaphragmatic breathing.

If you are in your first trimester, you can use POSITION 1, but if you are in your second or third trimesters, skip this position.

POSITION 1:
Lie down and elevate your feet with your hips and knees at 90 degrees. You could place your feet on the couch. Then, place your hands on your ribs and inhale until you feel them expand to about 80 to 90 percent capacity. Once you inhale, hold your breath briefly. Then slowly release the air and feel your ribs close and return to a resting position. Wait a few seconds, and then repeat. Spend 3 to 5 minutes focusing on your breath and the full expansion of your ribs.

POSITION 2:

If you are in your twentieth week of pregnancy or beyond, this is an ideal position. Sit on your bed with your head and upper body elevated 30 degrees. You can stack pillows or use bigger and firmer pillows. You can add a pillow under your knees, if that is comfortable.

Then, complete the same exercise from Position 1. Place your hands on your ribs and inhale until you feel them expand to about 80 to 90 percent capacity. Once you inhale, hold your breath briefly. Then slowly release the air and feel your ribs return to a contracted position. Wait a few seconds, and then repeat. Try to make the exhale longer than the inhale. Spend 3 to 5 minutes focusing on your breath and the full expansion of your ribs.

POSITION 3:

Sitting in a chair or practicing your breath while driving is also a great option. As you inhale, you should feel your back expand into the seat or chair. This position is a great way to get feedback that you are getting more of a 360-degree breathing pattern.

You can try this on an exercise ball as well. This will engage your core as you practice breathing. It's a full-body experience! Some women prefer to do breathing exercises while standing, but beware of your shoulders. Are they hiking up? Keep your shoulders relaxed and feel your ribs and belly for full expansion.

HELPFUL BREATHING HINTS

- If you are having trouble with beginning a diaphragmatic breath, begin by sniffing. When you sniff, you are taking the first step to a correct inhale for a diaphragmatic breath. As you inhale, the diaphragm contracts, opening the lungs for more air. This action creates downward pressure on the abdominal area. You will feel your belly expand slightly. Continue the inhale from your sniff to feel the belly and ribs expand in all directions. This sensation is called 360-degree rib expansion.

- Start with a sniff and then move to a bigger inhale. This takes practice! Don't expect to master it on the first try. Relax and practice breathing.

- Sometimes people visualize breathing with colors: inhale the blue and breathe out the red. Others say, "Smell the roses and blow out the candles." Even others create mantras that are relaxing and empowering. The process of breathing well is preparing you to deliver well and live well.

- Start today. Start now. Diaphragmatic breathing is a simple but powerful step that anyone can take to improve their muscle coordination, mindfulness, and overall well-being. Spend time discovering the right time of day and the right mantra to help you make this a habit.

As with every other *One Simple Step Today* chapter, my goal is to give you a simple step that fits into your daily routine to help prepare you for pregnancy. Diaphragmatic breathing should not feel like another

"To Do" on your list. Instead, work it into your day. When you wake up in the morning, rather that reaching for your phone, pile up a few pillows and begin the day with your breathing exercises. You are already in position! Try to make it a habit to breathe consciously before your reach for your phone.

This is a great habit for any person, whether pregnant or not. Begin your day with mindfulness rather than screen time. Take a moment in the early morning light to center your mind and to focus on your body. Become aware of any tightness or discomfort that presents itself as you breathe in the morning. As the weeks continue and your baby grows, that minor "tightness" can become "muscle tension." Then, if not corrected, that muscle tension turns to "pain" and can progress to "constant pain." If you can address the issue when it's only "tightness," you can save yourself a lot of discomfort.

In addition to breathing in the morning, add diaphragmatic breathing to your nighttime routine. Once again, you are already in bed. This should not feel like an EXTRA thing to do. It should just become part of what you do to prepare for sleep. At night, take inventory of your body and how it feels. Breathe in and notice the parts of your body we discussed in Chapter 2. If you ever feel something out of the ordinary, make a note of it in your phone. As you keep a running list of notes, you will be prepared for your next doctor's appointment.

This habit has another important benefit. As you regularly train your body, you are also going to become better and better at listening to the muscles involved in delivery. Although many health professionals give the advice to "listen to your body," most of them never teach you how to do so. This is a formula for listening to your body.

Each day, you must pause and breathe and give all of your attention to the small changes happening to you. Make a note of those changes and address them with your doctor, midwife, physical therapist, and whoever is on your health team that supports you through this pregnancy.

As with everything in this guide, this is an introduction to these concepts. If this is very difficult, don't feel like you've failed. Many women need more detailed instruction one-on-one, which is why it is so important to see a women's health physical therapist who specializes in the pelvic floor. Additionally, I love to coach women so they can connect to their bodies, so let's set up a time to chat!

This kind of breathing is perfect training for delivery. You are beginning to control the muscle groups that will work together to deliver your baby.

Your *One Simple Step Today* is to begin to practice diaphragmatic breathing and choose several times in your day to incorporate it as your daily routine. It's such a healthy habit!

Journal & Reflection

WHEN I SLOW DOWN AND DO DIAPHRAGMATIC BREATHING, I FEEL:

_____

_____

_____

_____

_____

I WANT TO PRACTICE DIAPHRAGMATIC BREATHING DURING THESE TIMES OF DAY OR SITUATIONS:

_____

_____

_____

_____

_____

_____

_____

_____

DAY 3 VIDEO LINK

Diaphragmatic Breathing
www.onesimplestep.today/bookvideos

BECOMING
MORE IN TUNE
WITH THE
PELVIC FLOOR
CAN IMPACT
SO MANY
aspects of life.

DAY 4

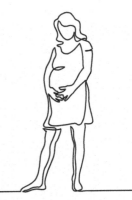

PELVIC FLOOR MOVEMENTS

What is your pelvic floor and why is it so important during your pregnancy? Your pelvic floor is a bowl of muscles from the pubic bone to the tailbone. These muscles are dynamic, full of energy and provide support for your bladder, womb, and bowel. They also play a big part in controlling leakage and aid in sexual enjoyment. These muscles are often overlooked, but during pregnancy, it is critical that women know how to control these muscles in order to prepare for a vaginal delivery.

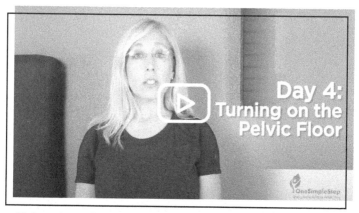

Click to view video or view full link listing at the end of the chapter.

Some estimate that as many as half of women are doing these pelvic floor contractions incorrectly. In one study, 1 out of 6 women weren't able to do a pelvic floor contraction correctly on the first attempt. However, after brief instruction, 78% of these women were able to learn how to do a pelvic floor contraction correctly.[v] This means some women will need to consult a physical therapist for further coaching. Do not be embarrassed if you need further assistance with this movement. You can reach out to me as well for a coaching session. It's very common to ask for help! Try the cues below as your *One Simple Step Today*.

THERE ARE THREE POSITIONS OF THE PELVIC FLOOR:

- Tight or Elevated or Lifted
- Resting/Neutral
- Lengthened and Lowered

In the last chapter, your *One Simple Step* was to begin regular diaphragmatic breathing. In this chapter, we are going to build on that habit. As you take your deep, diaphragmatic breath, you are going to connect that breath with your pelvic floor. That's it; this is your *One Simple Step Today*! You will be learning how to coordinate your pelvic floor through contracting and relaxing. Not only will you be strengthening and controlling and relaxing the muscles needed for vaginal delivery, but you are also setting up your body for long-term health and stability.

The best way I know to teach you how to perform a pelvic floor contraction is to give you multiple cues and allow you to choose the one that best helps you to visualize and control these muscles. These cues are specifically for learning the first position of the pelvic floor: contracting.

Remember after each contraction or lift of the pelvic floor to allow your pelvic floor to return to a rested position. Staying in contracted or tightened position for a long time can lead to pelvic pain and tension.

Let's begin working on these pelvic floor contractions. You may also know them as Kegel exercises.

CUE #1: STOP THE FLOW OF URINE, MIDSTREAM (COMMON, BUT NOT MY FAVORITE!)

This is a commonly used cue to help women know how to tighten their pelvic floor and relax it. When you are using the restroom, use the muscles in your pelvic floor to stop the flow of urine. This is the tightened or elevated position I was referring to.

Then, release the flow of urine and feel your pelvic floor relax. The only problem with this cue is that it should not be used regularly. Stop the flow of urine only rarely, at most once a week, as it is not recommended to use this as an ongoing exercise. The problem that can result is an inability to fully empty the bladder. So, use this cue to identify the sensation so that you are isolating the pelvic floor muscles.

If you cannot stop the flow of urine, don't worry; there are other ways to identify the muscles. Often, women who have weakness in the pelvic floor muscles cannot stop the flow of urine.

CUE #2: WASHCLOTH IN A CHAIR

Place a rolled-up wash cloth in a chair and sit on it, like sitting on a saddle. Sit up tall. With your underwear on, try to lift AWAY from the washcloth. Notice the ability to lift or contract your pelvic floor. Please understand that it is not squeezing the gluteus maximus or your butt! In this cue, you can feel the movement of your pelvic floor upward, away from the washcloth.

CUE #3: THE BLUEBERRY METHOD

Imagine you have placed a blueberry in a chair. Visualize picking up that blueberry with your vagina. Sit tall, tighten and then release as you envision picking up the blueberry off the surface and then releasing it.

CUE #4: THE JELLYFISH MOTION

Think of the motion a jellyfish makes as it swims through the water. Try to make that same motion with your pelvic floor. If you can visualize how a jellyfish swims, you can imagine this is how the deep muscles of your body work together. There is a smooth lifting upward and a gentle relaxation downward. One up, one down, and so on.

CUE #5: SQUEEZE AROUND THE PENIS DURING SEX

You can try this with your partner, or you can imagine what it feels like. This cue helps you to really isolate the muscles. Often the contraction of the pelvic floor muscles is small, so don't get discouraged if your partner cannot feel you squeeze your pelvic floor. As an added bonus, another purpose of the pelvic floor muscles is to assist in sexual function and enjoyment. Stronger and more coordinated pelvic floor contractions can contribute to ability to achieve an orgasm as well.

CUE #6: ICE COLD POOL

Pretend you are walking into a very cold pool of water. As you enter the water, your pelvic floor naturally draws upward. Feel the natural lift that comes from your body's automatic reaction.

CUE #7: HAND ON YOUR UNDERWEAR

Although this is similar to the "Washcloth in a Chair," my clients have told me that it helps to FEEL rather than just SEE the pelvic floor contraction. With your underwear on, place your hand gently on your vulva, the area outside of the vagina. Then, lift away from your hand. Engage only the pelvic floor to lift and then relax the muscles touching your hand.

CUE #8: EXERCISE BALL

Sit on an exercise ball, if you have one. Perform a pelvic floor contraction as you sit. Now, for a more advanced maneuver, lean forward, with more pressure on the urethra and clitoris, as you contract. In this position, when you perform your pelvic floor contraction, you should feel the vagina tightening. Lean backward toward the tailbone and feel a rectal contraction. In the middle, everything draws up and in. Engage the vagina and rectum to contract together. If you don't have an exercise ball, you can do this on a chair, but sometimes it's easier to feel the movement on an exercise ball.

Your *One Simple Step Today* is to practice the different ways to contract and relax the pelvic floor muscles. See which one helps you the most. Laying down is easier than sitting, and sitting is easier than standing when trying to turn on these muscles.

DAY 4 VIDEO LINK

Turning on the Pelvic Floor
www.onesimplestep.today/bookvideos

Journal & Reflection

WOW, I HAVE LEARNED A LOT ABOUT MY PELVIC FLOOR:

_____

_____

_____

_____

_____

THE BEST CUE FOR A PELVIC FLOOR CONTRACTION FOR ME IS:

_____

_____

_____

_____

_____

_____

_____

_____

_____

DON'T FORGET YOUR
pelvic floor!

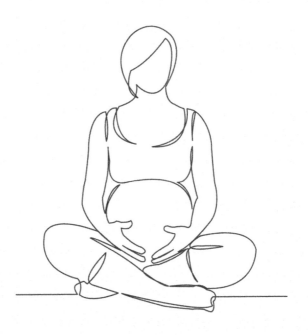

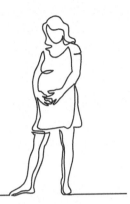

DAY 5

ZIPPING UP AND LENGTHENING THE PELVIC FLOOR

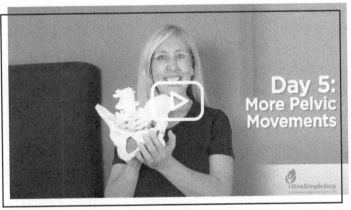

Day 5:
More Pelvic Movements

OneSimpleStep

Click to view video or view full link listing at the end of the chapter.

Great job! If you tried each of those cues in order to engage your pelvic floor, you have given yourself a gift. You have learned how to connect with your pelvic floor, specifically by lifting, elevating, and tightening. Not only that, but you have begun a journey toward a strong and healthy core, and your body will thank you for years to come.

Let's continue building on these skills by putting together your diaphragmatic breath with your pelvic floor contraction. This motion can be called, "ZIPPING UP." In the same way that a zipper pulls your jeans close to your body and keeps them closed, this motion will pull your pelvic floor close to your body to engage your muscles from the bottom up.

First, take a good inhale and feel the pelvic floor lower a little bit (this position is lowering or lengthening). Then exhale, like you are blowing out a candle. As you exhale, contract the pelvic floor and lift the pubic bone slightly. Engage your pelvic floor muscles and transverse abdominals to pull that entire area upward. Even when you are pregnant, you can see your belly button slide in toward your back. Place your fingers on your transverse abdominus, just inside the ASIS. If you forget where this is, refer back to Day 1!

ZIP UP STEPS

1. Inhale and feel the pelvic floor lower slightly (lengthening or lowering position).

2. Exhale and draw up your pelvic floor and continue the "zip up" to include lifting the pubic bone (tightening, lifting, and elevating position).

3. Feel the transverse abdominus muscle tighten ("like a corset").

4. Inhale again to feel the pelvic floor relax and lower.

You can practice this motion while you are lying down or while you are sitting. To try it in a resting position, use these steps:

1. Lie down with pillows behind your back so your upper body is at a 30-degree angle.

2. Prop your knees with two pillows.

3. Inhale and feel the pelvic floor lengthening.

4. Exhale and tighten or lift the pelvic floor.

5. As you exhale and feel the pelvic floor pull upward, lift the pubic bone slightly.

Remember not to hold your breath. Once you exhale completely, continue breathing. Keep practicing until the motion of ZIPPING UP is something you can do easily. ZIPPING UP is the motion you will need to keep your core strong as the baby grows. Your core is turned on and muscles are contracting.

ZIPPING UP is not a continuous state you want to remain in. It's a tool for helping manage the abdominal and pelvic pressure you may feel when doing various activities of life. Remember to inhale and relax the pelvic floor and abdominals after the activity.

In upcoming chapters, we will learn to ZIP UP in certain daily situations as the baby grows. Don't worry about that yet, though! Your *One Simple Step Today* is to coordinate your diaphragmatic breathing with your pelvic floor movement to gain more awareness of your body. There are multiple places and times you can practice this. Practice in the morning while still in bed. Practice on an exercise ball while you work or watch TV.

LENGTHENING THE PELVIC FLOOR

We've gone through how to connect and engage your pelvic floor by moving from resting to tightening, elevating, and lifting.

Now we are going to focus specifically on lengthening and lowering the pelvic floor. This practice is different from the lengthening we talked about when you inhale during diaphragmatic breathing.

It is important to clarify that this lengthening happens during the EXHALE versus the INHALE of diaphragmatic breathing...

because lengthening the pelvic floor has a different purpose...

and those two purposes are...

pooping and vaginal delivery.

What it is NOT:

- bearing down
- turning red in the face
- Valsalva (think about heavy weightlifters holding their breath)

What it IS:

- extending your pelvic floor
- on an exhale breath
- with your throat open!

How do you poop when a little constipated? Often, it is pushing as hard as you can to get that poop out. The risk here is pelvic organ prolapse. You're pushing the poop through a restricted hole, your anus. You're creating pressure in your core system, which puts you at risk for damage. It's restricted because the pelvic floor is tight.

So, what is a better way to poop and prepare for vaginal delivery? Lengthening the pelvic floor!

You can practice when you poop. Breathing while pooping helps you feel the same sensation because that motion of pushing is what you will feel in your pelvic floor during a vaginal delivery. Your job during delivery is to lengthen the pelvic floor to provide an opening for the baby to be born. The uterus actually does the pushing. Exhale and visually see the pelvic floor lowering toward the toilet water, staying mindful of your pelvic floor.

As with other muscles in our body, the pelvic floor will begin strengthening as you practice. As you work on contracting, lengthening, ZIPPING UP, diaphragmatic breathing, and exhaling with exertion, you are giving your body a gift. You are working on coordinating your muscles for your delivery. Bonus, you didn't have to go to a gym or even leave your bedroom/bathroom. You can work out in the comfort of your home and at your own leisure. Just add these movements as a regular part of your day so when the day comes to go to the hospital and deliver the baby, you will be ready!

Your *One Simple Step Today* is to practice your pelvic floor movements. Think about how you poop and remember to practice lengthening the pelvic floor with exhale next time you poop. Don't worry, it may take practice!

DAY 5 VIDEO LINK

More Pelvic Movements
www.onesimplestep.today/bookvideos

Journal & Reflection

THESE ARE SOME WAYS IN MY DAILY LIFE THAT I CAN BEGIN CONNECTING TO MY PELVIC FLOOR AND ZIP UP:

_____

_____

_____

_____

_____

_____

_____

_____

_____

_____

_____

_____

_____

_____

_____

_____

HOW YOU STAND CAN AND WILL IMPACT
how you feel.

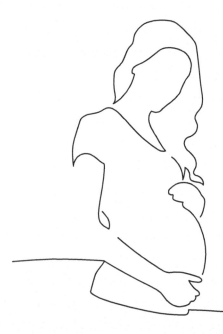

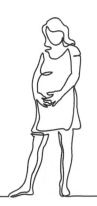

DAY 6

POSTURE

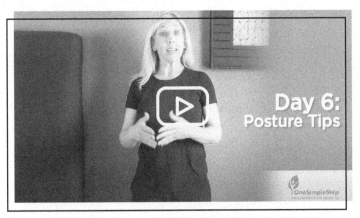

Day 6:
Posture Tips

Click to view video or view full link listing at the end of the chapter.

Living well includes moving well, so this chapter will focus on strong, healthy movements that can easily be incorporated into your day. Strong, healthy movements begin with proper alignment. If we are not in correct alignment, our body will produce pressure in places where we don't want it.

Let's try to simplify what it means to have good posture by starting at the top. Let's start with our head.

Think of your head as a bowling ball and your neck as a stick. Now picture that heavy ball is perched on top of the stick. If the ball is too far forward, it strains the stick. The result can be tension in the neck and shoulder region.

The easiest way to make sure your head is in alignment is to act like someone is pulling up on your head by your ponytail. That motion stacks your head on top of your shoulders, your ribs on top of your pelvis, and your knees over your feet.

Think about the time you spend on your phone, with your head in a forward posture. The average weight of the head is about ten pounds, but as you lean forward that weight becomes more burdensome and the strain on your body increases. Misalignment also causes tightness in the neck and shoulders.

Stop a moment and do *One Simple Step Today* to improve your health. Stand in front of a mirror and turn to the side. Notice your posture. Is your head stacked on top of your shoulders or are you leaning forward? If it's hard to see your posture, ask a friend to take your profile picture. They need to take a full-body profile picture so you can see your natural standing posture.

After analyzing the picture, change your posture by pretending someone is pulling up on your ponytail. Keep your shoulders relaxed but straighten your spine and lift your head without arching your back.

Now, look in the mirror or have a friend take your picture again. Compare the two photos. What do you see?

Although your posture is unique to you, there are two common postures that cause strain during pregnancy. One is the "Pregnant Hang" posture and the other is the "Rounded Back" posture. These postures are also known as an anterior pelvic tilt or posterior pelvic tilt.

PREGNANT HANG POSTURE
(Anterior pelvic tilt)

When we are out of alignment in the "Pregnant Hang" posture, we generally see:

- Arched spine
- Boobs upward
- Knees locked
- Back muscles are overworked or strained

This posture makes you appear to be hanging on at the hips. It may have been the way you posed for pictures to make your belly look rounder.

Try this position as you look in the mirror. Feel the strain it places on your back. Also, while in this position, try to take a deep, diaphragmatic breath. It is impossible to get a full diaphragmatic breath. If you try to tighten the pelvic floor, you will feel that it is almost impossible as well.

Ideally, we want to stack the ribs on top or over the pelvis. This position is known as a neutral pelvic tilt. Try to look in the mirror. Again, how does it feel? Take a deep breath and tighten the pelvic floor muscles. Do you feel the difference? Which position makes it easier to breathe?

ROUNDED BACK POSTURE (POSTERIOR PELVIC TILT)

The second common misalignment is the "Rounded Back" where your spine is curved in the shape of a "C." In this posture, we generally see:

- Rounded spine
- Butt tucked and tight
- Boobs downward
- Rounded shoulders
- Head forward
- Knees locked

Once again, this posture is not optimal because it prevents deep breathing and puts strain on your joints. Try this position and feel how shallow your breathing becomes.

In an optimal alignment, our head is stacked on top of our shoulders and ribs are directly over the hips. The hips are in line with the knees and knees are directly over the feet.

Another cue that can improve your standing posture is to pay attention to the weight distribution on your feet. Think of your feet as a tripod with the three parts being the big toe, little toe, and heel. Weight should be even on all three parts. If not, you are placing strain on your knees, hips, or back.

Once your weight is evenly distributed and your ponytail is pulled upward, check your hips. Hips should be in a neutral position, not forward-tilted, backward-tilted, or jutting to the side in order to hold your toddler. To find your neutral hip positioning, simply make sure your ASIS and pubic bone line up flat. Another way is to look in a mirror, practicing both the anterior and posterior pelvic tilt dramatically to figure out the neutral position between them. For some people it's easier to start lying on the floor to feel the movement against the floor.

Now that we've discussed posture, it's important to realize that no one can live in this posture at all times. We have to be able to move and function freely! Don't feel like you are a paralyzed robot. You will not break if you move into a variety of positions, but you can be empowered to move with awareness.

Now that you are in tune with a strong and correct posture, you can make adjustments to deal with aches, discomfort, or pain. As always, if you need one-on-one help, ask for it! A physical therapist may be able to help set you up for a win.

Don't forget to take your *One Simple Step Today*: check out your posture. Use a mirror, or even have someone take a picture of you. For a more accurate check, ask someone to take a picture of you when you're not aware of it. In doing this, you can become more mindful of how you typically stand. It can be very eye opening!

DAY 6 VIDEO LINK

Posture
www.onesimplestep.today/bookvideos

Journal & Reflection

AFTER LOOKING AT MYSELF, I CAN DESCRIBE MY TYPICAL POSTURE AS:

_____

_____

_____

_____

_____

I WANT TO BEGIN IMPROVING THIS ASPECT OF MY POSTURE:

_____

_____

_____

_____

_____

_____

_____

_____

POSTURE + CORE
+ MOVEMENT

=

increased freedom

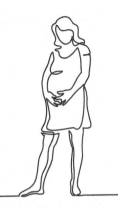

DAY 7

FUNCTIONAL MOVEMENT

Congratulations! You have discovered what it feels like to be more aware of your posture. Let's keep going by taking posture awareness into daily movements.

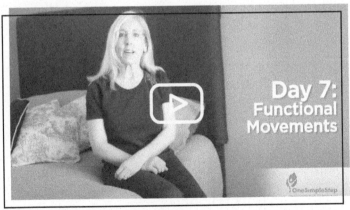

Day 7:
Functional
Movements

Click to view video or view full link listing at the end of the chapter.

Posture does not only refer to our positioning when we are still. Our bodies are dynamic, moving from position to position throughout the day. In order to reduce pain and strain, we need the body awareness, strength, and coordination that centers around our core as we move.

Let's discuss five important, repetitive movements that you can master in order to give you more freedom and keep your body more supported during pregnancy.

1. SIT TO STAND

We have all seen a pregnant woman struggle to stand up while carrying the weight of a bowling ball in her belly. In order to avoid the typical "belly first" approach to standing, try the following steps:

First, scoot forward in the chair. Next, align your nose over your toes. This means you will lean forward slightly. Use your arms as support and exhale with exertion. As you blow out that air, remember to ZIP UP, and then stand with strength. Whenever you stand, remember your core. Don't leave your core on the floor! Standing with strength means bringing your core muscles, which include your pelvic floor, with you as you move upward. Remember the bottom of the box! (It's helpful for me to think of the TA muscles as a corset for these movements.)

2. LIE DOWN IN THE BED

First, sit on the bed with both legs perpendicular to the bed. Then, exhale with exertion to prepare to move. Next, bring both legs up onto the bed and move your shoulders downward in one flowing movement. Remember to move to side-lying first. Keep your knees together during the entire effort.

3. SLEEPING POSITION

After working with pregnant women for two decades, I know that finding the right position during sleep is a critical part of overall happiness during this journey. First, let me assure you that you will need plenty of pillows! Many women love their pregnancy pillow (a long, snake-like pillow that can support different parts of the body). After 20 weeks, side sleeping is the optimal sleeping position. In order to be comfortable and aligned, I recommend placing two pillows between your knees that extends to your ankles. These two pillows are placed strategically to keep your back and pelvis aligned.

In addition, as you enter the second trimester, you will likely need a pillow under your belly, supporting the weight of the baby. You can add a fourth pillow under your arm. I also suggest adding a hand towel rolled up like a burrito, inside the base of your pillow to support your neck. A pillow behind your back is also very helpful so all your weight isn't on your shoulders.

4. TURN OVER IN BED

Turning from one side to another can become a challenge as your baby grows and the weeks pass. The safest way to turn from one side to another is to begin by exhaling with exertion. ZIP UP and squeeze the pillow between your knees. You can also squeeze your ankles together as this helps to maintain your alignment. In one single flowing movement, engage your core and turn. Do not leave one leg behind, as this puts strain on your back and pelvis.

5. LIFTING

As your pregnancy enters the second and third trimester, you must reduce the amount of lifting you are doing on a daily basis. I know this can be difficult! I was pregnant while caring for a toddler, and he did not understand that Mama should not carry him all day.

Even if you cannot eliminate lifting completely, see if you can reduce it. Be creative! For example, instead of lifting your toddler from the ground, you can sit on the couch and ask him or her to climb into your lap. If you are pregnant with your second or third child, this is good training for when the baby arrives.

For everyday activities such as lifting your gym bag, work bag, laundry basket, or groceries, try to place items in strategic locations so they do not have to be lifted from the ground. Reducing the stress and strain on your body will make life easier, and your body will be happier as the pregnancy progresses.

When you must lift, start with your feet shoulder-width apart. Keep your chest up and bend your knees. As you lift upward, exhale with exertion and ZIP UP! If it is a challenge to squat, hold onto a doorknob or even place a chair under you as you squat. It's not a bad idea to do at least one squat per day during your pregnancy (as long as your doctor has not limited this movement due to breech position or high-risk pregnancy).

A second way to lift, if you don't have pain or pressure, is to hinge at the hips and reach downward with a flat back. Depending on how far along you are in your pregnancy and how flexible you are, it can be a good option if you are picking up a lightweight object like a toy or small purse or unloading the dishwasher. This movement is similar to a deadlift. Inhale as you hinge at the hips, and exhale as you lift.

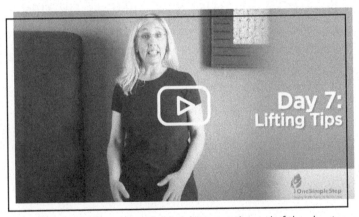

Click to view video or view full link listing at the end of the chapter.

Let me add a few other tips about movement that are important things to remember as you progress in your pregnancy.

SITTING IN THE OFFICE

When you are working or sitting for long periods of time, remember that this is not optimal during pregnancy. Our bodies are not made to sit for longer than 30 minutes. During pregnancy, it is even more critical that you stand often. If you are in a meeting, sit near the door so you can exit to use the bathroom or walk around as needed. If you are in a conference or at church, sit near the back of the room. Scan each room and find the best seat for a quick walk.

I also recommend an exercise ball as a chair, even during pregnancy. Sitting on an exercise ball engages your core and allows you to move your pelvis throughout the day.

COOKING AND OTHER STANDING ACTIVITIES

Just as our bodies are not meant to sit still for long periods of time, we are also not meant to stay on our feet for hours and hours. If you are a teacher, doctor, nurse, cashier, mom, or a worker in any other profession that could require long periods of standing, I recommend you take frequent breaks. Now that you know how to stand with proper alignment, you are better equipped, but you still need to take breaks. For example, if you are waiting for water to boil, sit down. If you are teaching a class, use chairs, stools, and desks as places to rest. While at home, sit down to take a phone call.

AVOID ONE-LEGGED ACTIVITIES

No, I am not referring to hopping. During pregnancy, sit down on the bed to put on your underwear and pants. Then, stand once both legs are in. Also, don't cross your legs when you sit in a chair, not even at the ankles. By keeping both legs going in the same direction as much as possible, you will reduce the pressure on your pubic symphysis joint and prevent strain and pain.

Does this mean you have to give up all single leg exercises? It depends. If you're not having pain, continue. If you're having pain, then adjust what you're doing. Your body will talk to you; don't ignore it!

As your baby grows and your body changes, your center of gravity is changing week by week. If you can modify what you are doing now and make these small, simple changes early enough, you can keep your body in proper alignment.

Once again, it would be impossible to cover proper positioning for every move you make in a day. There are thousands of them! Julia Di Paola, a well-known physical therapist, says, "Your body will work best in the optimal alignment, where you breathe the best and have the rib expansion, but you can't live there. So, you have to have variety of movement. Start in neutral but connect in all movement patterns."

Today you have taken a step to becoming aware of alignment and misalignment in your body. You are creating new habitual patterns of moving that will serve you throughout your pregnancy and your entire life.

You have the power to be stronger if you are aware of your alignment and position and how you are moving through your day. These little changes don't have to weigh you down. These are things you are doing anyway. You already get into bed. Why not enter the bed in a way that supports your core? You already roll from side to side. Now you will keep your spine supported as you roll. Congratulations on creating new habits today. Your older self will thank you. Plus, if you are creating these habits in your first trimester, your third trimester self will thank you as well!

Your *One Simple Step Today* is to be aware of your movements. Is your body talking to you? Can you modify some activity and give your body relief?

DAY 7 VIDEO LINKS

Functional Movements
www.onesimplestep.today/bookvideos

Lifting
www.onesimplestep.today/bookvideos

Journal & Reflection

THESE ARE SOME MOVEMENTS THAT I DO MANY TIMES DURING MY DAY:

_____

_____

_____

_____

_____

THESE ACTIVITIES CAUSE ME DISCOMFORT, SO I WILL TRY TO MODIFY HOW I COMPLETE THESE MOVEMENTS:

_____

_____

_____

_____

_____

_____

_____

_____

PAIN IS COMMON.
PAIN SHOULD NOT
BE CONSIDERED
NORMAL.
PAIN SHOULD BE
ADDRESSED,
not ignored.

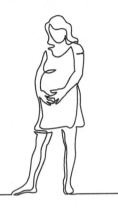

DAY 8

SIGNS, SYMPTOMS, COMMON COMPLAINTS OF PREGNANCY

You have taken so many simple steps each day as you go through this book! Congratulations on making it this far. You have begun to train your body to move with proper alignment, awareness, and mindful breathing. You have also started training your body to adapt to non-ideal positions through awareness of your core, pelvic floor, and back.

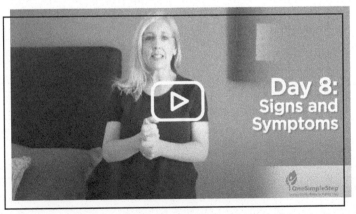

Day 8:
Signs and Symptoms

OneSimpleStep

Click to view video or view full link listing at the end of the chapter.

You have begun listening to your body and can identify specifically what you are feeling. As you listen, you may notice signs and symptoms that cause concern. Although this is not an exhaustive list of the many strange feelings you may experience during pregnancy, it can give you some information about when to STOP and consult your doctor immediately:

- Changes in vision or speech
- Headaches or fever
- Prolonged nausea and/or vomiting
- Changes in Baby's movement
- Spotting or bleeding
- Rapid swelling
- Urinary changes or pain
- Blood pressure of 140/90 mmHG or higher, or 10 mmHG above normal BP
- Anything that doesn't feel right

For any of the feelings above, make sure to contact your doctor or hospital. I cannot stress this enough. Make a phone call for reassurance and for safety. Err on the side of calling too many times, especially during your first pregnancy. If you need a phone call for peace of mind, make the phone call. Contacting your healthcare provider not only can improve your physical health, but receiving reassurance improves your mental and emotional health as well. Don't overlook the mental, emotional, and spiritual aspects of your health, especially during pregnancy.

If you are listening to your body and you have pain or strain, this chapter is to help you understand what you are feeling and what steps to take to modify your movements and communicate exactly what you are feeling to those on your birthing team.

While we are on the subject of your birthing team, let's discuss some of the people who can help you on this journey. First, you need an OB/GYN who is overseeing your care. (You may also have a secondary doctor or OB/GYN if you have an at-risk pregnancy.) Next, you may want to enlist the support of a physical therapist who specializes in women's health. Schedule 2 to 3 appointments with your physical therapist throughout the pregnancy and at least one visit six weeks after delivery. If you are not sure where to find the right physical therapist for you, try ChoosePT.com and look for someone who is trained in women's health.

You may also find it helpful to hire a midwife and/or doula. A midwife has medical training, works with the doctor, and focuses on the delivery of the baby and care of the mother. A doula is a non-medically trained professional who provides continuous emotional, physical, and informational support to a mother before and after labor.

In addition, consider enlisting the help of a mental health professional who specializes in prenatal and postpartum health.

COMMON COMPLAINTS
Below are seven common complaints I have dealt with

in my twenty years in women's health physical therapy. With each complaint, I am offering tips for resolving each specific type of discomfort. As always, if pain continues or if it is limiting how you walk or function, discuss with your doctor and advocate for yourself. If it is dismissed as normal during pregnancy, continue to ask for a full evaluation by a women's health physical therapist. Speak up for yourself now in pregnancy, during delivery, and the rest of your life!

1. ROUND LIGAMENT PAIN

Round ligament pain is usually a sharp pain in one or both sides of your lower abdominals. You might feel this abdominal pain when you are sitting in a chair and begin to stand. The pain you feel is the ligament that supports the uterus. That ligament is being stretched as the baby grows. If you feel this type of pain:

- Slow down your movement, so you are not standing quickly and haphazardly. Rather, stand up slowly and deliberately. This will help your core support you and take some strain off the round ligament.

- Rest.

- ZIP UP before you stand.

- If it continues, even as you stand slowly, contact a physical therapist or chiropractor. They can perform a massage on your ligament to relieve the pain.

2. PUBIC SYMPHYSIS JOINT PAIN OR SYMPHYSIS PUBIC DYSFUNCTION (SPD)

Also known as "lightning crotch," pubic symphysis pain occurs in 1 in 5 pregnancies. During pregnancy, the pubic symphysis opens and expands in order to make more space for the baby to descend. This gradual opening can cause mild discomfort to debilitating pain. Pain appears more commonly with single leg activities, such as putting on pants or climbing stairs. If you begin to feel this type of pain:

- Avoid single leg activities as much as possible.

- Pretend you are wearing a tight pencil skirt. This will force you to keep your knees together when walking, exiting a car, climbing into bed, or rolling over in bed.

- If you make an appointment with a physical therapist, you can get a stabilization belt to help as well.

- Avoid cross your legs at the knees or at the ankles, as this puts more strain on the pubic symphysis.

3. SACROILIAC JOINT PAIN

Commonly referred to as SI pain, you can feel this discomfort in the dimples of your lower back. My patients have often described it to me as feeling like their back is locked or a feeling of instability in their lower back.

- Once again, try to keep your knees together and avoid one-legged activities.

- If small modifications in movement don't work, you will need to make an appointment with a physical therapist who can help you modify movements more specifically, give you a stabilization belt, and prescribe specific exercises for your specific needs.

4. SCIATICA

Sciatica refers to back pain caused by a pressure on the sciatic nerve. This is a large nerve that runs from the lower back down the back of each leg. As the baby grows, there's more pressure on the sciatic nerve, that nerve is pinched. Women often describe it as pain that feels like it's deep in their butt. It can cause shooting pain down your leg.

- Use a tennis ball, racquet ball, or some type of firm but squishy ball that can be used to roll deep into the butt. Sit on the ball or place it up against the wall. This movement can relieve pressure on the nerve and allow your muscle to relax.

- "Nerve glides" can be helpful in relieving pain. Think about your nerves that run from the back and continue down the leg. Sometimes, they get "hung up." Nerves need to move freely. Nerve glides are like flossing the nerve.

  - Sit on a chair.

  - Straighten the knee.

  - Pump the ankle up/down 10 times.

  - You should feel a gentle stretch.

5. UTI – URINARY TRACT INFECTION

If you experience back pain below the ribs, you could have a UTI, which is common during pregnancy. This is a referred pain pattern from the kidneys to the low back region. Referred pain patterns occur when you feel pain somewhere, but not at the source of the pain. UTI may be accompanied by a burning sensation while peeing or increased frequency in the amount of times you need to go to the restroom. Your urine may appear dark or have an odor.

If you are concerned that you might have a UTI, schedule an appointment with your doctor immediately because you may need antibiotics to treat it.

6. INCONTINENCE OR LEAKAGE OF URINE OR STOOL

These symptoms indicate that there is a weakness or a lack of coordination of the pelvic floor muscles. Refer back to chapter three whenever the smallest amount of leakage begins. If you can address minor leakage, you can prevent a bigger pressure management problem. Never ignore it! It is not normal to leak during pregnancy or even during an exercise class, or anytime in your life. It's not a normal consequence of pregnancy or aging!

- Practice pelvic floor contractions.

- ZIP UP before standing, sitting, and rolling in bed.

- If you cannot modify your movement, make an appointment with a women's health physical therapist. You can talk to your doctor at your next appointment about your desire to see a women's health physical therapist. Address this problem before delivery; don't ignore symptoms.

7. PROLAPSE – PELVIC FLOOR PROLAPSE OR VAGINAL PRESSURE

If you ever feel like something is falling down into your vagina, this feeling should be taken seriously.

Women describe it as feeling like they are sitting on a small ball. Pelvic organ prolapse is when the uterus, rectum, or bladder drop down into the vaginal cavity. Whenever you feel pressure in your vagina, make an appointment with your doctor. Discuss this at your next appointment with your healthcare provider . This is a great reason to see a pelvic floor physical therapist during your pregnancy. It's important that this symptom is not ignored. Delaying treatment until after delivery may intensify the symptom.

8. DIASTISIS RECTUS ABDOMINIS – SEPARATION OF RECTUS ABDOMINUS

Almost 100 percent of all pregnant women will experience diastasis recti, or separation of the abdominal muscles by the end of third trimester.[vi] Truly this is the amazing way the body adapts to the uterus growing 500 times its original size. This condition causes a doming of your belly that bulges out whenever you lift or do something strenuous, or even standing up. This usually occurs at, below, or above the belly button.

It is important to modify or decrease the intensity of whatever activity you are doing. The goal is to minimize the advancement of the diastasis recti. ZIPPING UP and using your pelvic floor and abdominals together will help provide more support as you go throughout your day.

For many women, this condition resolves itself naturally in the first 3 to 6 months postpartum. However, as always, a pelvic floor physical therapist can provide appropriate exercises to strengthen your core and ways to not aggravate your symptoms.

9. CONSTIPATION

Did you know that your digestive system slows down so you can gain more nutrients from your food during pregnancy? This miracle that allows the baby to receive a maximum amount of nutrients causes approximately 25 to 50 percent of pregnant women to experience constipation.

- Drink a cup of hot water first thing in the morning—even before your coffee or tea.

- Use a step stool under your feet as you sit on the toilet. This stool places your knees higher than your hips to open up the pelvic floor.

- Add fiber to your diet. I recommend blueberries, coconut water, and prune juice.

- Increase fiber slowly and record it so you are aware of what you are taking in.

- Don't bear down with each bowel movement. Work on exhaling and lengthening your pelvic floor with pooping.

- Try to walk every day, even 10 minutes can make a difference.

If you try all these natural things and nothing works, communicate with your doctor. If you ignore constipation, you can get pelvic organ prolapse or hemorrhoids that will follow you into postpartum. Please do not use just ANY over-the-counter stool softener. You must discuss with your doctor before taking any medication during pregnancy and while breastfeeding.

10. DIZZINESS OR NAUSEA WHEN LYING ON YOUR BACK

After 20 weeks of pregnancy, you should not lie down on your back for long periods of time.[vii] Try to limit the time to 2-3 minutes. When you are pregnant, your uterus can press on your inferior vena cava (the large vessel that carries blood from your lower body up to your heart), affecting your blood supply.[viii] If you feel dizzy or lightheaded, be sure to change positions. However, some women find that they subconsciously roll onto their backs at night, even though they begin the night on their side. Rather than stress about this, do the best you can. When you wake up or go to the bathroom, use pillows to prop and support you in a side-lying position.

- If laying on your back, elevate your trunk from the waist up by 30 degrees with pillows or a wedge cushion.

- Roll onto your side. Use pillows behind your back to encourage you to stay on your side.

- If you are feeling dizzy while lying on the table at the doctor's office, tell your healthcare provider that you need to sit up or change positions.

I recommend that every pregnant woman include a physical therapist on her birthing team. A full evaluation by a women's health physical therapist can make sure you have a more comfortable pregnancy and uncover other contributing factors to unnecessary pain. I hope this chapter introduced you to common complaints of pain during pregnancy, so you feel equipped to be prepared in any situation.

I also hope this chapter helped you to expand your idea of the types of people who should be a part of this journey with you. Every person is unique, and every pregnancy will have joys and challenges. In addition to your doctor, physical therapists, midwives, doulas, massage therapists, chiropractors, and mental health coaches can guide you through this journey and help you improve your overall health for years to come.

Your *One Simple Step Today* is to consider your birth team. If you are having pain, contact the right medical professional for help. Even before you experience pain, make a plan for a birthing team who will support you on your journey! Remember, it's a great option to see a pelvic floor physical therapist 1 to 2 times during your second and third trimester, as well as postpartum.

DAY 8 VIDEO LINK

Signs and Symptoms
www.onesimplestep.today/bookvideos

Journal & Reflection

AT MY NEXT DOCTOR'S APPOINTMENT, I NEED TO DISCUSS THESE SYMPTOMS OR CONCERNS:

_____

_____

_____

_____

_____

_____

_____

_____

_____

_____

_____

_____

_____

_____

_____

PEOPLE I WOULD LIKE TO BE PART OF MY BIRTHING TEAM IN PREGNANCY, DELIVERY, AND POSTPARTUM:

_____

_____

_____

_____

_____

_____

_____

_____

_____

_____

_____

_____

_____

_____

Preparation
IN PREGNANCY
HAS A BIG IMPACT
ON DELIVERY DAY.

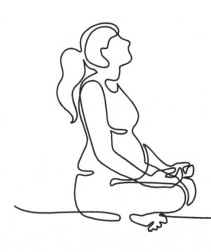

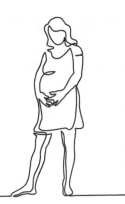

DAY 9

MINDSET

The right mindset or overall mental attitude can affect your pregnancy experience, your baby, and your delivery. Never before has your mindset been more important! Your *One Simple Step Today* is to get into the right frame of mind in order to give your body and mind the best environment for a successful delivery.

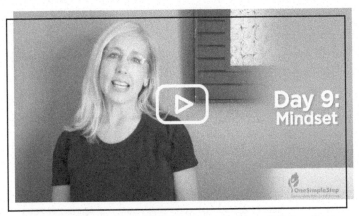

Day 9:
Mindset

Click to view video or view full link listing at the end of the chapter.

We are going to use 3 Simple Steps to achieve a positive mindset: Practice. Plan. Prepare.

FIRST SIMPLE STEP: PRACTICE

I always tell my moms-to-be, "The delivery room should feel comfortable because of your preparation." In other words, it's important to practice everything that you will be using for birth before you are in the delivery room. You do not just wake up and run a marathon. You practice! You train every day in order to give yourself a successful race day.

So, in this chapter, we are going to begin practicing the following things on a regular basis in order to feel comfortable in the delivery room and to have a successful delivery day.

PRACTICE MINDFULNESS

The definition of mindfulness is "being in the present moment and not judging it or trying to change it." You will need to have the ability to be completely present and living in the moment during delivery. You have already begun a mindfulness routine as you practice diaphragmatic breathing and pelvic floor movements, but now you can put it all together for one whole mind-body experience.

Start your day with breathing and mindfulness. Center yourself and let go of the worries that typically flood your mind. When it is time to give birth to your baby, you are going to do this as well. You are going to devote your focus completely to the task at hand. Walk into the hospital for delivery and leave the world behind you. Those other things can wait. Right now, you are going to be present in this important moment.

PRACTICE LISTENING TO SOOTHING MUSIC TO RELAX

What music helps you to be relaxed and calm? Or what music helps motivate you during the contractions? Music can be a powerful force for your mood, so use it. Try different playlists and various artists to see which ones help you to experience a peaceful state of mind.

Remember that you can bring devices to the delivery room. Many women put in their cordless earbuds, just like they are running a race. Others bring speakers or just use their phones. However you choose to play your music, spend some time practicing your breathing and mindfulness with the music you will use that day.

PRACTICE USING ESSENTIAL OILS TO DISSIPATE ANXIETY AND FEAR

There are ways essential oils can help you during this time. First, smells have a powerful calming effect on the body. Using lavender can help your body relax. Many women diffuse oils in the delivery room. So, practice it now. If you feel yourself becoming stressed, diffuse various oils to see which one helps you the most. Practice active relaxation with essential oils.

Research and prepare now to know which oils you like and dislike. Lavender, peppermint, and orange are just a few essential oils commonly used by women in delivery.

If your hospital doesn't allow you to diffuse essential oils during your delivery, you have other options. Bring cotton balls or gauze pads and put a few drops of oil on it. Place it near your nose so you can inhale and feel the benefits of the essential oil.

Another option is to dilute the essential oil with a carrier oil, such as fractionated coconut oil, and place in a roller bottle. Your birth partner can gently massage your shoulders or feet as you desire.

PRACTICE PERINEAL MASSAGE

Perineal massage is a good way to prepare the perineum to stretch and reduce tearing. In your third trimester, discuss perineal massage with your doctor to see if it would be recommended to begin to prepare the tissues and provide some elasticity with anticipation of vaginal delivery.

Perineal massage is a daily stretch for approximately 5 minutes, completed by yourself or with your partner's assistance. You will gently insert your finger inside the vaginal opening and begin stretching in a U-shaped movement from three o'clock to nine o'clock. This information is to provide an introduction to this IDEA, so please get more information before beginning perineal massage. More instruction can be provided by a pelvic floor physical therapist, a doula, or in a birthing class.[ix]

PRACTICE POSITIVITY WITH YOURSELF

Although your body is changing and life is changing at a rapid pace, it is important to focus on the positive as much as you can. Hold on to the big picture and keep the prize at the end in mind. Pregnancy and delivery can be beautiful in the midst of chaos, so focus on the beauty as much as possible.

Your body actually has a physical response to happiness that helps you in a vaginal delivery. As you focus on the positive and feel positive feelings, your body produces oxytocin. When the hormone oxytocin is released, your body speeds up the birthing process. Conversely, when you feel stressed, your body slows down the birthing process, due to cortisol hormone being released. So, positivity is not only a good mantra for happy living, but it is essential to childbirth!

Remember the following mantra when you need to change your mindset. First, "Pause and pivot." Second, tell yourself, "I can do this." As you change your behavior and your thoughts, congratulate yourself by saying, "I am doing this." You may find other statements that are more helpful for you. Begin using these mantras before your delivery.

PRACTICE POSITIVITY WITH YOUR BABY
Hopefully, you have been speaking positive words to your baby throughout the pregnancy. Continue into delivery. I know one mom who said, "You come when you're ready!" Then, after the due date, she changed it to "It's time to be born!"

PRACTICE POSITIVITY WITH YOUR PARTNER
Once you have learned how to produce a positive mental state alone, it's time to practice positivity with your birth partner. Since you will probably not be alone in the delivery room, you must practice like it's real life!

If your birth partner is a friend or family member, it's still a good idea to spend time together and discuss different scenarios that you may encounter in the delivery room. Expressing and talking about what helps relax and calm you can be beneficial before you deliver your baby.

A suggestion for a way couples can practice this is with "Couch Time Together." My husband, Pete, and I have been using this strategy for years, and it's a great habit to begin as you are becoming parents. After we eat dinner, we sit on the couch and reconnect. We process our day and just enjoy one another! Even though the kids are making noise and the house is not completely silent, we find our moment of peace together.

When you are in the middle of the craziness of delivery, it's important that you two know how to be together. You need to know what you can do together that relaxes you. This is not a place for stressful conversations or arguing. The only goal of this time is relaxation. Communicate with your partner about topics that relax you. Figure out how to be intimate and connected in the middle of chaos.

Like a quarterback who has to stay relaxed and focused even as linebackers are coming toward him, you and your spouse can practice relaxing in the middle of it all.

When I was in labor with my first child, the contractions got particularly intense. Pete and I started talking about the different ways we add and subtract big numbers. What a random topic! It wasn't rocket science. We were not solving world problems. We were just talking about something that kept my mind off the contractions and helped me relax.

As the two of you go through delivery together, you will become more powerful and more focused. You will gain another level of centering energy and will create a powerful bond between you. It is the job of your birth partner to learn what is relaxing to you and be ready to create that kind of environment as much as possible.

During this private, intimate time that you are practicing, don't bring any anger or dissension. The delivery room is no place for it! Remember, stress slows down the birthing process, so this is about creating a space for focused relaxation.

Even romantic ways of touching and kissing can release oxytocin. The feeling of love can relax the cervix, so communicate with your partner if there are ways to hold your hand, massage your shoulders, or kiss your forehead. Whatever makes you feel loved and safe is a good thing!

But you may not want to be touched, and that is okay too. Take a moment and reflect on how you are feeling, what will take away fear, anxiety, stress, and pain.

Isn't it a great feeling to know that your *One Simple Step Today* is to figure out how to feel happy and positive? What a fantastic assignment! Use mindfulness, music, essential oils, and breathing to get into a state where your body is relaxed enough for delivery.

SECOND SIMPLE STEP: PLAN

Making a plan goes hand in hand with relaxation. Some women need a more detailed plan, as that is their personality, while others feel bogged down with too much planning. There is no perfect guide, but I suggest that you discuss the various possibilities that can happen in labor and delivery and have a general idea of your preferences. You cannot truly PLAN the entire delivery because there are too many variables.

Dr. Joel M. Evans, a leader in the field of Women's Health and a speaker at the 2020 Birthing Summit said it well when he said, "Don't come in with a rigid birth plan. It doesn't work." He goes on to explain that rigidity in this fluid process can actually prevent your best outcome.

Instead, make your peace with all the various possibilities that could happen in labor. Mentally accept that you might have a vaginal delivery or a cesarean delivery. Remember the goal is a healthy mom and a healthy baby. You may have a preference about many things, but they are just preferences. You have not failed if the process looks different than what you imagined.

However, you can share your birth preferences with everyone on your birthing team. They are here to help you in every way possible! From your birthing class instructor to your physical therapist to your doctors and nurses, speak up and let them know what you prefer. Having a voice helps you relax and move confidently in the direction you desire. Having a long-term vision for the ultimate outcome will keep you relaxed if the plan changes.

I have created a Birth Preparation Guide that you may find helpful as you plan. Take time to complete the questions and reflect on them. Planning now can greatly impact your birth experience.
Go to: www.onesimplestep.today/birthguide

THIRD SIMPLE STEP: PREPARE

Now that you have made your plan and you have practiced what you will do in the delivery room, it's time to make some key preparations. Once again, based on your own personality, it's important to prepare enough to feel safe and secure.

Taking a birthing class is very helpful for both you and your birthing partner. There's so much information about what to expect. Often, you get the opportunity to practice different labor positions. This is also a great time to ask more questions and learn more.

Some preparations to consider are:

- Taking a hospital tour
- Packing bags for you and your birthing partner
- Scheduling a birthing class (virtual or in person)
- Creating a text group on your birthing partner's phone for updates to your loved ones
- Installing the car seat
- Gathering clothing in sizes preemie, newborn, and 0 to 3 months

- Stocking up on diapers in those same sizes
- Preparing postpartum essentials like pads, mesh underwear, nursing bra, spray bottle, etc.

There are more extensive lists you can download online in order to prepare for delivery, but as a mother of three, I promise you do not need to check everything off every list. Prepare enough to feel comfortable and relaxed and then congratulate yourself for taking that one simple step!

Prepare to know the difference between Braxton-Hicks contractions and true labor.

One question I hear from my first-time mothers is, "How do I know if the contractions are labor-related or if they are just Braxton-Hicks contractions?"

My first answer is, "You are going to breathe through them the same way, so don't worry about it too much." However, here are three ways to know the difference:

1. True labor comes in regular intervals. Braxton-Hicks contractions have no pattern.

2. True labor is felt all the way through your abdomen and often into your back. Braxton-Hicks contractions are only in one part of your abdomen.

3. Rest, a warm bath, and fluid intake will not stop labor.

These three things will generally take care of Braxton-Hicks contractions. Many moms have found it helpful to record all the contractions, including Braxton-Hicks on a downloadable app. A simple search will provide you with options that fit your needs.

Of course, as always, when you are unsure, call your doctor or go to the hospital. Many first-time mothers go to the hospital for Braxton-Hicks contractions, and it eases their concerns. Some women experience a lot of mild contractions before labor, while some do not. My encouragement to you is to breathe and drink water and relax as much as you can. These three steps will guide you.

Another preparation step is to stay hydrated. The fluid that you consume 24 to 48 hours prior to delivery affects the elasticity of the pelvic floor. This can help reduce tearing. IV fluids may be needed and helpful in delivery, but they cannot replace how hydrated you are as you enter delivery. This is why it's extra important to stay hydrated in your third trimester!

Sometimes, you can prepare extensively and still there will be hiccups. When I was eight months pregnant, I had to practice flexibility when my OB/GYN closed her practice. My birth plan was definitely disrupted. I had to grieve the loss and then quickly pivot.

The next step required changing to a larger practice and meeting all the potential doctors that would be delivering my child. This required a new goal and steps to meet this in a time-sensitive situation. I couldn't become paralyzed by frustration.

I was able to meet all the OBs in the practice prior to my delivery. I felt comfortable going into my delivery. After all was said and done, I met my baby boy and smiled through tears as all the difficulty was worth it!

However, if you are having trouble pivoting or focusing on the positive, you are not alone. One in 5 women deal with anxiety and fear during pregnancy.[x] It can help to meet with a mental health professional to deal with the emotions you are feeling. Some of it can be attributed to the hormonal changes in your body, but it is also related to the newness of this whole experience. Get the help you need to bring a relaxed mental attitude to your pregnancy, labor, and delivery.

You may not have to deal with your doctor closing his or her practice, but there will likely be hiccups. Resolve today to handle those with a positive attitude in order to stay focused on the long-term goal.

This chapter covered many items, so you may want to take more than one day to work on Practice, Plan, and Prepare. Your *One Simple Step Today* is to pick out 3 items that you want to focus on in the next week. You may want to come back to this chapter and review it periodically in the time leading up to your delivery.

DAY 9 VIDEO LINK

Mindset
www.onesimplestep.today/bookvideos

Journal & Reflection

THINGS I NEED TO PRACTICE:

_____

_____

_____

_____

_____

THINGS I NEED TO PLAN:

_____

_____

_____

_____

_____

THINGS I NEED TO PREPARE:

_____

_____

_____

_____

LET'S
do this!

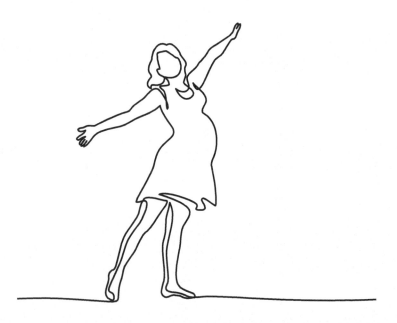

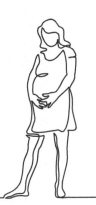

DAY 10

LABOR AND DELIVERY

The day is here! You have done the preparation. You have learned about your body and how to breathe through a variety of situations. Now, it is time to breathe through labor and delivery.

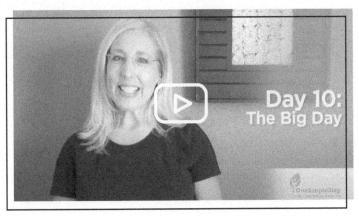

Day 10:
The Big Day

Click to view video or view full link listing at the end of the chapter.

Although every labor and delivery story is different and every woman's body is unique, there are certain aspects that are universal. Remember, women have been giving birth in their homes, by themselves, for years. Throughout time, women have done this. You can do this! Your body was made for it, so relax and know that you are prepared and ready for labor.

In fact, the most important thing you can do is relax and open the pelvic floor. Your breathing, positivity, and focus are all geared toward that one end:

OPEN THE PELVIC FLOOR.

Remember that fear and worry will slow down the progression of labor by tightening the pelvic floor. As you breathe through contractions, stay connected to your body and allow relaxation to guide you.

This is true whether you are induced or go into labor naturally. It is true whether you are rushing to the hospital or waiting for your water to break.

Relax.

Allow the pelvic floor to open.

Take the breathing techniques you have been practicing in the morning and in the evening into the delivery room. Breathe through your contractions, not only to manage the pain, but also to speed the process of delivery. Remember, when you feel safe and secure, your body produces oxytocin, which helps the baby progress through birth. Your calming presence can help your baby now, and it is great preparation for the calming presence you will need to breastfeed, rock a crying baby, hug a toddler, play with a young child, and even assure your teenager that they are okay.

In fact, you are already becoming a great mother. Even as you read this book, I want to congratulate you on taking great care of your baby today. You are already a fantastic mom! You are loving your child enough to take time to learn about what he or she needs, and that is a sign of an extraordinary parent. *Your One Simple Step Today* is learning how to help yourself and your baby through the process of labor and delivery.

Another thing that will guide you is the fact that you have made peace with all birthing possibilities.

I have had two deliveries and one adoption, and none of them went exactly according to plan. In fact, I had to be induced twice and my husband was more disappointed than I was. He wanted to rush to the hospital, like they do in the movies, and he felt robbed of that excitement!

However, when you get to the hospital or even if you are having a home birth, keep your eyes focused on the prize ahead. In a short period of time, your baby will be here.

LABOR AND DELIVERY

Once you arrive with your birth team, you will continue to do the things you have prepared to do. You are bringing your breathing, relaxation, and positive attitude into the delivery room. The only new addition now is the fact that doctors and nurses will be giving you cues. Listen to their instruction and ask questions when you are unsure.

Ask questions like:

- Can I move to a different position?
- Can I kneel?
- Can I try squatting or lying on my side?
- Can I use a birthing ball?
- Can I labor in the shower?

Try to stay in an upright position and walk as long as you're able. Having gravity on your side will help you progress and the baby to drop lower.

Maybe laboring in the shower is an option. Time spent standing or walking or sitting or leaning over the elevated bed allows your baby to press down on the cervix, assisting the laboring to progress.

Of course, if you are restricted for various reasons to the bed, as I was in my labor, adjust to changes and keep the whole picture in mind!

Some labor and birthing positions are:

- Sitting on a birthing ball
- Propped with pillows behind you
- Side-lying
- Squatting or kneeling
- On hands and knees

- Leaning over raised bed
- Walking
- Traditional/Lithotomy (on back)

You can even meet with a physical therapist in your third trimester to find out which birthing position is optimal for your pelvic floor. A PT can use a biofeedback machine that allows you to see when your pelvic floor is contracted or relaxed. A high number means the pelvic floor is contracted or less relaxed. A lower number means the pelvic floor is very relaxed. Your goal during delivery is to have a very low number, so a physical therapist can provide various positions to try in order to get the lowest number possible. The added knowledge of how your pelvic floor relaxes can be so helpful.

As you move into your second stage of labor, it is critical to listen to your nurses, midwife and doctors. They might ask you to stop pushing at times or change positions at times. The nurse is trying to prevent tears, prevent hemorrhoids, make sure the baby is getting enough oxygen, and more. Listen to your nurse carefully.

Before you know it, you will be holding your new baby girl or baby boy and all the preparation will be worth it!

C -SECTION TIPS

If you have a planned or unplanned cesarean delivery, many of the things we have discussed can be very helpful. Essential oils, breathing and music can still be part of your amazing delivery process.

You can still ask for skin-on-skin immediately after the birth of your baby. You can speak up for your preferences as well. Staying well informed as to the steps in the procedure is important too. Ask questions. Depending on the situation, your birth partner may need to take a bigger role as your advocate.

Tips for your birth partner to remember in the case of an emergency c-section is to bring essential oils, phone/camera and ear buds.

AFTER DELIVERY

After delivery of your baby, your body will immediately feel different. You have just removed a large amount of volume from your abdomen, and you now have to reconnect with your new body, even as you are taking time to connect with your baby. The third stage in labor is delivering the placenta. You will have postpartum contractions to breathe through, so as you are breathing, take those full diaphragmatic breaths in order to help your body begin to heal. These full breaths help you to reconnect to your body.

You should expect to have post-delivery contractions, which is helping your uterus returning to its normal size. These can be painful, but they are very helpful. You may notice them occurring with breastfeeding too, as there is hormone release. They are often called, "afterbirth pains," or "involution," and they can last for up to one week after delivery. A heating pad can help. It also helps if you use the bathroom regularly to reduce the effect of these types of cramps. Your nurse in the hospital will be there to help you through these pains. Although uncomfortable, take time to be grateful that this is the way your body returns the uterus to its original size.

Please note that women who have had c-section deliveries will also have these uterine contractions. It can be very surprising, especially if it was a planned cesarean delivery. This may be a completely new feeling if you didn't experience contractions prior to delivery.

Finally, once you have delivered your baby and breathed through postpartum contractions, you will also need to breathe through your first bowel movement after delivery. Drink some hot water and ask for a stool softener. Begin to eat fibrous foods after delivery and stay hydrated. It might feel a little bit scary to use the restroom after birth. Everything feels sensitive, but you can do this. You have been breathing and relaxing for months. Make sure to apply those principles here.

Another helpful tip is to use a foot stool and rest your feet on it. You simply want your knees to be higher than your hips in order to be in the optimal position. This is important because it allows the pelvic floor muscles to relax. You want the pelvic floor to work with you for a successful first poop!

You will probably receive a peri bottle at the hospital. Using this "squirt bottle" will allow you to avoid wiping the perineum after peeing and pooping. It is a gentler way to keep this area clean. When you do use toilet paper, remember to dab instead of rub.

Lochia is postpartum bleeding. It may be heavy for a week to 10 days. For many women it may become lighter but may last for 4 to 6 weeks postpartum. Every woman is different. If you have concerns that the bleeding is heavier than expected, please make sure to call your doctor. As always, it's best to discuss and bring up any concerns rather than wait until your 6-week visit.

Before you are discharged from the hospital, ask any questions. It's also helpful to have your birth partner take notes because you will be receiving so much information about healing and taking care of yourself as well as your baby.

Labor and delivery will be unique for you, but after taking a birthing class and preparation, you will be ready. You are ready for the adventure that leads to the birth of your child. Congratulations on taking this *One Simple Step Today* to prepare for the journey!

DAY 10 VIDEO LINK

The Big Day
www.onesimplestep.today/bookvideos

Journal & Reflection

MY IDEAL DELIVERY AND BIRTH STORY WOULD BE:

_____

_____

_____

_____

_____

_____

_____

_____

_____

_____

_____

_____

_____

_____

_____

_____

_____

Journal & Reflection

HOW I HOPE TO ADAPT TO CHANGES THAT MAY OCCUR IN MY BIRTH EXPERIENCE :

_____

_____

_____

_____

_____

_____

_____

_____

_____

_____

_____

_____

_____

_____

_____

_____

DELIVERY DETAILS I NEED TO DISCUSS WITH MY HUSBAND OR BIRTH PARTNER:

_____

_____

_____

_____

_____

_____

_____

THINGS I NEED TO RESEARCH MORE BEFORE DELIVERY:

_____

_____

_____

_____

_____

_____

THE
IMPORTANCE OF
rest and healing
FOR MOM
CANNOT BE
OVERLOOKED
IN THE
4TH TRIMESTER.

DAY 11

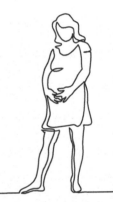

YOUR POSTPARTUM PLAN

The first twelve weeks after giving birth is often referred to as "The Fourth Trimester." We call it this because the baby still loves being treated like he or she is in the womb. Your little angel likes to feel the tight squeeze of a swaddle and hear swishing sounds as if inside the womb. However, the fourth trimester is also important to you as the mama! This is a time of healing and recovery as your body is going through as many changes as it went through during the previous three trimesters, all while taking care of a newborn baby.

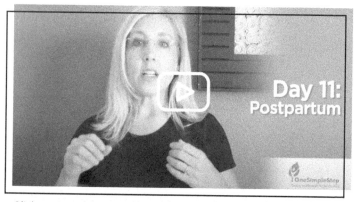

Click to view video or view full link listing at the end of the chapter.

In 1975, childbirth educator Shelia Kitzinger argued that moms need a lot of care in the weeks following birth. She said, "There is a fourth trimester to pregnancy, and we neglect it at our peril." There are now so many ways for a mom to be supported during this time, however women often do not reach for help and support. Don't try to do this alone.

While most women are very well supported during the first three trimesters, seeing a doctor every month and then increasing to every week and receiving attention from multiple professionals, they often feel alone immediately after birth. It doesn't have to be this way, though! You can make a postpartum plan to make sure you are preparing yourself to heal well and heal for life. Remember, the term postpartum means EVERYTHING AFTER BIRTH. Technically, the rest of your life is "postpartum," so let's make sure you are set up for success!

My first piece of advice about your postpartum plan

is to assemble a good team. Just as you assembled a fantastic prenatal team, you can enlist the help of others as you enter a time of healing. Of course, I am not suggesting that you will only need help for 12 weeks. It took nine months for your body to do what it needed to do to make this baby. I think you need nine to 12 months for your body to heal completely.

On a traditional medical tract, you will see your OB/GYN after six weeks and he or she will often say, "Everything looks great. You have the green light to return to life, exercise, and sex!" However, there is so much more happening in your life after the baby arrives. Pregnancy and delivery have left their marks on you, and it takes time to heal. Additionally, there are physical and emotional needs along with a life-change that is different for every woman.

My goal is to educate you and give you the steps to healing. I want you to have a pelvic physical therapist as your friend in all of this, so you don't have to go through it alone.

Before we begin the section on healing, it's important to examine other cultures to realize that women around the world are given more ample time to heal than here in the United States. Our family lived in China for three years, where it is a tradition that the mom and baby stay at home, resting for the first 30 days. For 30 days, new mothers rest at home and the world is kept at a distance. It is common in multiple other cultures to designate a period of time when the expectations for the new mother are absolutely minimal.

Compare that to what happens here in the United States. Women are shopping at Target two weeks after the baby is born. They are trying to call, e-mail, clean, work, and do it all as soon as possible. I am going to give you some important steps you can take in order to allow your body to heal well. The first one is to plan for a time of healing for your body.

HEALING STEP #1: DESIGNATE A TIME FOR RESTORATION.

Before you even go to the hospital, make a plan with your spouse or partner for a number of weeks when you will focus on resting, healing, and caring for your baby. During this time, you will do whatever you can to keep your level of work to a minimum. This time will be a gift to yourself and your new baby. Your focus will be entirely on recovering and bonding with your baby. Just feed yourself and your baby. There may be days where getting a shower marks the day as successful! Nothing else. Lower your expectations. Don't feel guilty about a dirty house. No need to apologize for rest and healing time.

- Writing thank you notes can wait. Enlist the help of your partner or a relative to write them for you.

- Cooking can wait. Use meals that were frozen prior to delivery or ask for friends to provide meals.

- Dirty clothes can wait. Laundry is a lot of lifting and bending, causing stress to your body. Ask for help.

It is time to focus on your baby, although it's easy to multitask while feeding your newborn. Lower your expectations for what you need to produce.

What if you had been in a motorcycle accident and you had a wound on your leg that was visible to the world? Since the world could see your wound, they would tell you to stay in bed and allow your body to heal. However, your wound is hidden, so the world is not telling you to stay in bed. Healing is important for all wounds, especially internal wounds.

Another tip, especially for healing after c-section delivery is try to stand taller each day. It's easy to guard incision and stand bent over. Unintentionally, doing this can cause additional tightness in the healing of your abdominal incision. Breathing and gradually standing taller can be helpful!

The pelvic floor, the C-section incision, and even the lining of the uterus where the placenta (the size of a plate) was attached needs time to heal like a burn. All of these wounds shouldn't be minimized or overlooked. Healing takes at least 6 weeks. You can look and feel great, but don't be fooled into overdoing it!

I think you will be surprised how well most people will react to your boundaries. If you tell them from the beginning that you are taking a specific number of weeks to heal, they will applaud you! They will work around your wishes. It is a great first step to setting boundaries you will need as a parent.

HEALING STEP #2: EAT THE GOOD STUFF FIRST.

Your body does an amazing job at healing, if you give it what it needs. What does your body need?

- Good nutrition
- Rest
- Minimal stress

While I am not a nutritionist and you can find plenty of resources about what to eat during pregnancy and after giving birth, I do have a very important piece of advice to keep your nutrition plan simple. Just eat the good stuff first. This is not a time for dieting. Of course, just like during pregnancy, if you are breastfeeding, you will need extra calories and you will have some cravings. However, eat whole foods and drink your water first. Don't start with the donuts. Fill your fridge with whole foods—vegetables, fruits, and protein—and begin with those. Food is medicine! As it turns out, your mama was right. You do need to eat your veggies before you have dessert!

We have to be realistic too! Consider a peanut butter and jelly sandwich on whole wheat bread as an easy thing to grab. String cheese, hard boiled eggs, and nuts are easy options, too. Often bland foods are helpful, including soups and broths. Make a list before you go into the hospital of foods you would like stocked in your house. Even consider this as part of your postpartum prep list.

HEALING STEP #3: CONTINUE DIAPHRAGMATIC BREATHING AND MINDFULNESS ABOUT YOUR POSTURE.

In this book, you have learned about diaphragmatic breathing, and you have made it a part of your day. It is one simple step toward mindful living. This time of breathing is a gift you can continue to give yourself. As you enter a time period that is devoted to your new baby, make sure to pause each day and give yourself some time. The moments when you place your hands on your ribs and belly and take those deep, cleansing breaths are just for you. Make time and space for yourself and your own health.

Also in this book, you have learned to be aware of your positioning. Keep that awareness and continue using it while breastfeeding and bottle-feeding. Just as you had to use pillows for correct sleeping position, use pillows to align your body and the baby's body for optimal positioning and balance. Check your shoulders; are they tense and guarded, or relaxed and soft? You will spend hours in this position. Make it comfortable and keep everything you need close to you!

Additionally, how are you carrying your baby? Often, we do the "mom hip hike." Avoid this method and keep your body balanced! Refer back to the posture chapter.

HEALING STEP #4: START WHERE YOU ARE NOW, NOT WHERE YOU WERE.

When you arrive home after the hospital, your body will undoubtedly talk to you. It will be giving you important feedback about what it can and cannot do. Commit today to listen carefully. This is your one simple step! Make a commitment before the baby arrives to be a good listener and honor what your body is telling you. Your exercise regimen can take a backseat to your need for rest. Once you have taken adequate time to rest, start slowly. Begin your new postpartum life without the expectation that you should immediately return to the level of exercise, sex, activity, and work you had before the baby arrived. You are starting fresh. Many women feel that their body becomes more stable, feels rested and ready to reintroduce exercise at the two-month postpartum mark. Even smarter an idea is waiting to return to running until three months postpartum.

Start slow, use diaphragmatic breathing, and reconnect to your pelvic floor again. You are in a new place. Begin with short walks. Remember the concepts we discussed in this guide for pregnancy and core and ZIP UP. Carry this new knowledge into your postpartum healing time. Make note of how your body feels.

Even if you feel great, you need time to heal. Don't rush yourself and pay for the consequences of being overzealous in returning to cardio exercise.

Wounds need six weeks to heal. Focus on healing. Even

at six weeks, the cesarean incision has not regained its full strength.

Ask to see your pelvic floor physical therapist at the six-week mark, the same as with your doctor. Even one visit to clear your pelvic floor and abdominals before returning to more exercise can prevent so many risks for future limitations and frustrations.

HEALING STEP #5: LET GO OF GUILT AND TAKE A NAP.

One of the best ways to speed up the healing process is by giving your body adequate sleep. But how does anyone accomplish this with a newborn? The answer is…you must prioritize your sleep over productivity. Let the laundry go. Let people help you. Let the text go unanswered. You just gave birth to a baby. Your body went through a major trauma. You need to sleep.

If you need to prepare your family members and friends now, go ahead. Let them know that you will not be answering messages for a while. Designate someone to take pictures and regularly send them to friends. Ask your spouse or partner to run interference. Whenever anyone asks, "Is there anything I can do for you?" give them something to do. Never say, "No, we are fine!" Let them bring you a meal, do some laundry, or run an errand. Give them a chore! Why not? You just had a baby.

While they are doing the chores, you take a nap. If sleep does not come easy, resting is beneficial too. What refuels, renews and refreshes you?

Another helpful tip to remember is diffusing lavender essential oil can be very calming and soothing

HEALING STEP #6: MAKE INTIMACY YOUR GOAL.

In a 2015 study, 85 percent of women report having some sort of discomfort with their first vaginal sex after childbirth. At three months postpartum, 45 percent of women report having discomfort. The number continues to drop each month after the baby is born. Even women who undergo a Cesarean section may report pain as they return to sex.[xi]

I do not give you these statistics to scare you but rather to prepare you and your spouse for what to expect when the baby arrives.

First, let's be clear: Pain during sex should never be ignored. Sex should not only be pain free, but it should be pleasurable for both of you!

One way to prepare your body for pleasurable sex is to complete scar massage to the perineal body, the area between the vaginal opening and anus. The goal is to decrease the sensitivity of the scar, increase the mobility of the tissues, and decrease overall pain. This is not only needed for sex but for sitting, exercising, bowel movements, and just living a pain-free life.

Your pelvic floor physical therapist can instruct you on the specifics of scar massage.

Another helpful tip in returning to sex is to use lubricant. You may have never dealt with dryness in the past but remember this is a new chapter. A great water-based lubricant is Slippery Stuff, which can be purchased on Amazon.

In order to receive the support you need to heal your body, you can ask your doctor for a referral at your six-week visit to see a pelvic floor physical therapist. By doing so, you can get support as you work to regain strength in your core and heal the layers of tissues that have been stressed through the delivery.

If you had a Cesarean section delivery, you can perform C-section scar massage after you've seen your doctor and the incision is closed and not infected. This step is important because seven layers of tissue have been cut and must heal so that you can wear clothing, move well, and even go to the bathroom normally. Once again, I would still recommend that you ask your doctor for a PT referral. This way, you have a professional on your side to help you heal.[xii]

Other common concerns in this postpartum time is incontinence or leakage of urine, stool, or gas. Also, don't ignore pelvic organ prolapse symptoms of heaviness in the pelvic area. Another symptom that should be addressed is diastasis recti, which often heals on its own, but if you are concerned, don't feel like your body has failed you! It just means you need a little bit more help to heal. A physical therapist specializing in women's health can be there for you.

Additionally, if you have questions for me and would like to talk, let's schedule a consult time!

CONGRATS, MAMA!

Congratulations on taking another simple step toward health! You have begun to plan for your postpartum healing even before delivery. Planning is the best way to ensure that you give your body the nutrition, rest, and support it needs. Remember that your abdominal muscles and pelvic floor have had pressure on them for nine months and that pressure was suddenly removed. It will take time to return to a new normal. Often, women report that they feel a big improvement in their body feeling stronger at two months postpartum. Cautiously move forward with exercise, and, as always, reach out for support!

Your body will continue to change throughout the fourth trimester and for the next year. Be patient with your body and listen to it. Address any concerns with professionals such as your health care provider, physical therapist, or mental health therapist. Continue to enlist the help of professionals along with a team of supportive friends and family members.

DAY 11 VIDEO LINK

Postpartum
www.onesimplestep.today/bookvideos

Journal & Reflection

THINGS THAT I NEED IN MY HOME FOR MY 4TH TRIMESTER:

_____

_____

_____

_____

_____

FOODS I WOULD LIKE TO HAVE IN MY HOME:

_____

_____

_____

_____

_____

WHO ARE THE PEOPLE THAT WILL HELP ME, AND WHAT TASKS CAN I DELEGATE TO THEM?

_____

_____

_____

Postscript

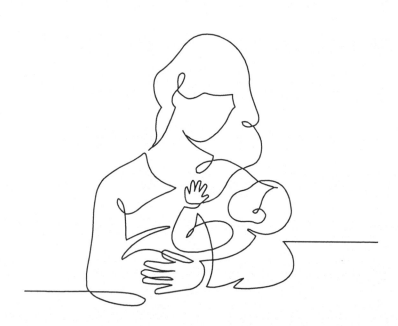

Dear New Mom:

You are incredible! You are beautiful. You are amazing. You will have moments you will never forget. You will shed tears. You will be tired. You will learn so much about yourself and your baby. You will love like you never knew you could love. You will have feelings you never thought you could experience. On the tough days, know that tomorrow is a new day to start over. On the lonely days, reach out for help. Celebrate the amazing moments. Take pictures to remember the messiness. Know your limits, and take care of yourself too, Mom! This journey of motherhood will not and cannot be perfect, but it will be beautiful. It is your journey!

From one mom to another mom,
Blessings and Love to you,
Heather Marra

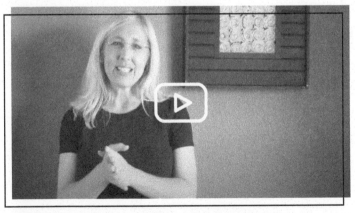

Click to view video or visit www.onesimplestep.today/pregnancyandbeyond/conclusion.

Journal & Reflection

LISTS AND QUESTIONS TO ORGANIZE MY THOUGHTS

THINGS I WANT TO BRING TO THE HOSPITAL:

_____

_____

_____

_____

_____

_____

THINGS I WANT TO BUY BEFORE GOING TO THE HOSPITAL:

_____

_____

_____

_____

_____

_____

THINGS I NEED TO DO BEFORE DELIVERY:

_____

_____

_____

_____

_____

_____

_____

PEOPLE TO CONTACT AFTER BABY IS BORN:

_____

_____

_____

_____

_____

_____

FIRST MEAL I WANT AFTER DELIVERY:

_____

_____

HIGHLIGHTS, MEMORIES, AND MOMENTS FROM MY 1ST TRIMESTER

_____

_____

_____

_____

_____

_____

_____

_____

_____

_____

_____

_____

_____

_____

_____

_____

_____

HIGHLIGHTS, MEMORIES, AND MOMENTS FROM MY 2ND TRIMESTER

_____

_____

_____

_____

_____

_____

_____

_____

_____

_____

_____

_____

_____

_____

_____

_____

HIGHLIGHTS, MEMORIES, AND MOMENTS FROM MY 3RD TRIMESTER

_____

_____

_____

_____

_____

_____

_____

_____

_____

_____

_____

_____

_____

_____

_____

THINGS I HAVE LEARNED THROUGH MY PREGNANCY AND WANT TO SHARE WITH OTHER PREGNANT MOMS:

_____

_____

_____

_____

_____

_____

_____

_____

_____

_____

_____

_____

_____

MY LIST OF: _____

QUESTIONS I HAVE:

THOUGHTS FOR MY BABY FROM ME, YOUR MOM:

_____

_____

_____

_____

_____

_____

_____

_____

_____

_____

_____

_____

_____

_____

_____

_____

ENDNOTES

[i] Gutke A, Boissonnault J, Brook G, Stuge B. The Severity and Impact of Pelvic Girdle Pain and Low-Back Pain in Pregnancy: A Multinational Study. J Womens Health (Larchmt). 2018;27(4):510-517. doi:10.1089/jwh.2017.6342

[ii] https://www.huffpost.com/entry/what-the-french-get-so-right-about-taking-care-of-new-moms_n_587d27b4e4b086022ca939c4

[iii] Woodley SJ, Lawrenson P, Boyle R, et al. Pelvic floor muscle training for preventing and treating urinary and faecal incontinence in antenatal and postnatal women. Cochrane Database Syst Rev. 2020;5(5):CD007471. Published 2020 May 6. doi:10.1002/14651858.CD007471.pub4

[iv] Minassian VA, Drutz HP, Al-Badr A. Urinary incontinence as a worldwide problem. Int J Gynaecol Obstet. 2003;82(3):327-338. doi:10.1016/s0020-7292(03)00220-0

[v] Henderson, Joseph Welles et al. "Can women correctly contract their pelvic floor muscles without formal instruction?." Female pelvic medicine & reconstructive surgery vol. 19,1 (2013): 8-12. doi:10.1097/SPV.0b013e31827ab9d0

[vi] Boissonnault JS, Blaschak MJ. Incidence of diastasis recti abdominis during the childbearing year. Phys Ther. 1988;68(7):1082-1086. doi:10.1093/ptj/68.7.1082

vii https://www.acog.org/clinical/clinical-guidance/committee-opinion/articles/2020/04/physical-activity-and-exercise-during-pregnancy-and-the-postpartum-period

viii Warland J. Back to basics: avoiding the supine position in pregnancy. J Physiol. 2017;595(4):1017-1018. doi:10.1113/JP273705

ix Ellington JE, Rizk B, Criso S (2017) Antenatal Perineal Massage Improves Women's Experience of Childbirth and Postpartum Recovery: A Review to Facilitate Provider and Patient Education on the Technique. J Womens Health, Issues Care 6:2. doi: 10.4172/2325-9795.1000266

x Fawcett EJ, Fairbrother N, Cox ML, White IR, Fawcett JM. The Prevalence of Anxiety Disorders During Pregnancy and the Postpartum Period: A Multivariate Bayesian Meta-Analysis. J Clin Psychiatry. 2019;80(4):18r12527. Published 2019 Jul 23. doi:10.4088/JCP.18r12527

xi McDonald EA, Gartland D, Small R, Brown SJ. Dyspareunia and childbirth: a prospective cohort study. BJOG. 2015;122(5):672-679. doi:10.1111/1471-0528.13263

xii Wasserman JB, Abraham K, Massery M, Chu J, Farrow A, Marcoux BC. Soft Tissue Mobilization Techniques Are Effective in Treating Chronic Pain Following Cesarean Section: A Multicenter Randomized Clinical Trial. J Womens Health Phys Therap. 2018;42(3);111-119. doi: 10.1097/JWH.0000000000000103

VIDEO LINKS

*All videos throughout this book are available at
www.onesimplestep.today/bookvideos.*

- Introduction to the Guide
- Day #1: What is the Pelvic Floor?
- Day #1: How Does the Pelvic Floor Move?
- Day #2: My Pelvic Bones
- Day #2: What Is the Core?
- Day #2: What's Down There?
- Day #3: Diaphragmatic Breathing
- Day #4: Turning on the Pelvic Floor
- Day #5: More Pelvic Movements
- Day #6: Posture
- Day #7: Functional Movements
- Day #7: Lifting
- Day #8: Signs and Symptoms
- Day #9: Mindset
- Day #10: The Big Day
- Day #11: Postpartum
- Postscript

ADDITIONAL RESOURCES

AMERICAN COLLEGE OF OBSTETRICIANS AND GYNECOLOGISTS (ACOG) FREQUENTLY ASKED QUESTION LINK:
https://www.acog.org/patient-resources/faqs

LOOKING FOR MORE INFORMATION ABOUT BIRTH, FINDING A DOULA, OR A VIRTUAL BIRTHING CLASS?
www.evidencebasedbirth.com

FIND A WOMEN'S HEALTH OR PELVIC FLOOR PHYSICAL THERAPIST NEAR YOU!
USA: www.aptapelvichealth.org
Canada: www.pelvichealthsoultions.ca

GENERAL PREGNANCY RESOURCE:
www.whattoexpect.com

POSTPARTUM SUPPORT INTERNATIONAL, FOR MENTAL HELP, SUPPORT AND RESOURCES DURING PREGNANCY AND POSTPARTUM:
www.postpartum.net
1-800-944-4773

ESSENTIAL OIL INFORMATION:
www.onesimpleoil.today

ACKNOWLEDGMENTS

This journey of writing was an adventure that I did not take alone. It would not have become a reality without the support of many friends and family.

My interest in PT began when I was in high school, and I observed my mom receiving physical therapy. Both my parents, Orie and Janie Ensz, encouraged me to pursue my dream of becoming a Physical Therapist. As I finished school, I became interested in pelvic health. My professor, Dr. Tom Sneed, urged me to begin immediately in this specialized area. He said, "The need for pelvic floor physical therapists is great. Begin now, and don't wait!" He was right!

Meredith Bauman and Karena Hayes, thank you for sharing your personal pregnancy experiences with me as this book unfolded. I am so excited as both of you embark on this journey of motherhood.

Thank you to Emily Osburne, Carey Phillips, Emma Sleeth, Krystal Cruz, and Rebecca Kurk, PT for all the input and editing that you each provided. Thank you to Heather Dauphiny for your beautiful artwork on the cover and interior design.

Joan Miller and Sarah Stonestreet, thank you for your encouragement, support, and listening ear.

I am grateful to Meredith Blase, who prayed for me, especially when I had lost my manuscript!

Pete, my husband, you are the love of my life. I enjoy living with an Enneagram 8, because as a Enneagram 1, we can get a lot of things accomplished! Thank you for believing in me.

Peter, Mateja, and Max, thank you for your patience, support, and involvement in this book project. You all have learned so much about the pelvic floor! I love being your mom and treasure the memories of both pregnancy and adoption with each one of you.

Nothing would be possible without the deep love of Jesus. My ultimate desire is that every woman experiences how deeply Jesus truly loves her.

ABOUT THE AUTHOR

With over 20 years of experience as a licensed Physical Therapist, Heather Marra continues to help women find healing and freedom in every aspect of life. She graduated from Southwest Baptist University, Bolivar, MO in 1998 with her Master's degree in Physical Therapy. She received additional training focused on women's health and pelvic floor physical therapy including CAPP-Pelvic (Certificate of Achievement in Pelvic Health Physical Therapy) from American Physical Therapy Association in 2008. Heather is a certified Pregnancy and Postpartum Corrective Exercise Specialist.

A highlight in Heather's career was working with Lilian Chen-Fortanasce, PT, in China as a teaching assistant for Maternal Rehabilitation Courses and presenting to the PT Rehab Team at the Chinese Olympic Center.

She has experienced the joy of two pregnancies as well as the adoption of her daughter from China.

Heather and her family lived in Shanghai, China for three years. They love exploring new cultural experiences, making friends from around the world and of course sampling international cuisine. Currently, they are residing in beautiful Colorado and enjoying the great outdoors with their dog, Courage.

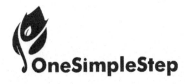

OneSimpleStep

WWW.ONESIMPLESTEP.TODAY

INSTAGRAM: @onesimplesteptoday

FACEBOOK: @onesimplesteptoday

TIKTOK: @onesimplestep

YOUTUBE: One Simple Step Today

TWITTER: @simpletoday

SPOTIFY: One Simple Step Today

LINKEDIN: https://www.linkedin.com/in/heathermarra/

EMAIL: heatherpt@onesimplestep.today

Made in USA - Kendallville, IN
1186631_9780578774824
10.27.2020 1036